D0225604

# Culture and AIDS

# Culture and AIDS

*Edited by*
Douglas A. Feldman

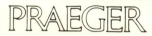

New York
Westport, Connecticut
London

**Library of Congress Cataloging-in-Publication Data**

Culture and AIDS / edited by Douglas A. Feldman.
      p.      cm.
  ISBN 0–275–93189–7 (alk. paper)
   1. AIDS (Disease)—Social aspects.  2. Ethnology.
 3. Anthropology.    I. Feldman, Douglas A.
RA644.A25C84    1990
362.1'969792—dc20       90–30003

Library of Congress Catalog Card Number: 90–30003
ISBN: 0–275–93189–7

First published in 1990

Praeger Publishers, One Madison Avenue, New York, NY 10010
An imprint of Greenwood Publishing Group, Inc.

Printed in the United States of America

∞

The paper used in this book complies with the
Permanent Paper Standard issued by the National
Information Standards Organization (Z39.48–1984).

10 9 8 7 6 5 4 3 2 1

# Contents

# Preface

This volume is not intended as an introduction to AIDS. There are several excellent books that could effectively serve that purpose. *Culture and AIDS* looks at AIDS as a cultural phenomenon. The way in which we as a species handle AIDS is a measure of our changing times, of our deepest fears, of our varying values, and of our collective aspirations. It is impossible to truly understand the role of AIDS in our lives unless we consider the social and cultural contexts of AIDS-related behavior. This volume is designed to clarify several key domains in AIDS and the social sciences. Nearly all of the chapters have been written by anthropologists, and they are representative of the interests of dozens of other anthropologists actively involved in AIDS research and activities.

I would like to thank the following individuals for their assistance in the development of this book: Dr. Richard Beach (University of Miami), Dr. Ralph Bolton (Pomona College), Mr. Carlos E. A. Coimbra, Jr. (Universidade de Brasilia), Dr. Paul Farmer (Harvard University), Dr. Norris G. Lang (University of Houston), Dr. William L. Leap (American University), Mr. Robert W. Lucero (PCS), Dr. Emilio Mantero-Atienza (University of Miami), Dr. Susan McCombie (University of Pennsylvania), Dr. Juliet Niehaus (New York University), Dr. Ronald J. Prineas (University of Miami), Dr. Michael D. Quam (Sangamon State University), Ms. Donna Sato (University of Miami), Dr. Frank Stitt (University of Miami), Dr. Christopher C. Taylor (University of Chicago), and Dr. Dooley Worth (Montefiore Hospital). This book is dedicated to the thousands of volunteers in AIDS-related community-based organizations worldwide who have given so generously of their time and effort in our relentless struggle against AIDS.

# Chapter One

## Introduction: Culture and AIDS

### Douglas A. Feldman

Our planet is a fragile ecosystem. The global warming effect, acid rain, toxic wastes, nuclear proliferation, overpopulation, major oil spills, ozone depletion, declining rain forests, animal and plant species extinction, rising crime rates and urban violence, gang warfare, poverty, increasing homelessness, and (until very recently) growing militarism are products of rapid technological, economic, and social change in a world undergoing major transformations. Advances in modern technology have resulted in not only the obvious improvements in our daily lives, but also brought unintended consequences leading to deleterious effects.

Acquired immunodeficiency syndrome (AIDS) is a good example of such a consequence leading to such an effect. It has rapidly emerged as a devastating global pandemic with major implications for the future vitality of humankind. While it is certain that we are much better equipped to develop treatments, possible vaccines, and prevention programs against AIDS on a global level today than we would have been, let's say, 50 years ago, it is equally certain that it is unlikely that AIDS could not have spread so rapidly without the development of modern commercial jet travel and the tremendous growth of urbanism in the Third World over the past few decades.

We do not know where and how AIDS originated, and perhaps we will never know. But let us briefly explore two possible scenarios. Scenario one: it is the 1950s and we are in a biological warfare laboratory in possibly the United States or the Soviet Union. An experimental retrovirus, later to be named human immunodeficiency virus, type one (HIV-1), is manufactured using an existing animal retrovirus as a model. Something goes terribly wrong. The virus escapes and gradually makes its way through sexual relations, infected needles, and blood transfusions to diverse at-risk populations in different parts of the world.

In scenario two, simian immunodeficiency virus (SIV) mutates into human immunodeficiency virus, type two (HIV–2), perhaps from blood contamination while skinning an infected monkey, possibly in a remote West African village many decades ago. This now human retrovirus rapidly evolves, and as it inadvertently spreads through sexual transmission into new tribal populations to the east, it takes on a more aggressive and more lethal character. By the late 1950s, the new virus HIV–1 has entered into the Belgian Congo (now Zaire) and perhaps elsewhere in central Africa. With the rise of urbanism and jet travel in central Africa, the virus spreads rapidly from city to city throughout central Africa, into Haiti, and among gay men in North America. By the late 1970s, about 4 percent of all sexually active gay men in San Francisco are infected. By the early 1980s, about 4 percent of all men and women in the central African nation of Burundi are similarly infected.

Perhaps there are other equally viable scenarios. One can always speculate. But speculation on the origins of AIDS has already caused much consternation, distress, and harm. As Paul Farmer discusses in this volume, early speculations that AIDS may have originated in Haiti had severely stigmatized the citizens of that country. Tourists stayed away from Haiti. Economic investments declined. Haitian-Americans found themselves increasingly losing their jobs. It is possible that the economic pressure caused by this fear of AIDS may have, at least in part, been responsible for the overthrow of the "Baby Doc" Duvalier regime in Haiti during the mid–1980s.

Current speculation that AIDS may have begun in Africa has also allowed anti-African bigotry to flourish. AIDS is blamed on Africans, or blamed on gays, or blamed on Haitians. AIDS is a stigmatized and stigmatizing disease and social phenomenon that is perceived to pollute everyone and everything.

The truth about the legitimacy of assigning blame, however, is quite the opposite. Retroviruses do not have morals. They move through human populations without conscious intent. If HIV–1 did originate somewhere in Africa, or North America, or Europe, or Asia, or elsewhere, it spread from person to person without anyone aware of its lethal direction. There is no blame to share for the early spread of the disease because no one is guilty.

In less than a decade, AIDS has become a truly global pandemic. In southwestern and northern Uganda, located in east Africa, half of all adults under 50 today are seropositive for HIV. The Ugandan extended family is under considerable stress as more and more children of parents with AIDS become orphaned. Husbands are mercilessly casting out from their homes their wives with AIDS, since the shame of their presumed infidelity is too much to bear. TASO, a self-help counseling group of concerned volunteers in Kampala, Uganda, helps persons with AIDS cope with the reality that they have the disease. They teach them about symptomatic HIV infection, allow them to explore their feelings about having this terrible disease, and instruct them on safer sex practices.

About 1,300 miles farther south, in Lusaka, Zambia, one in four adult men and women between 20 and 50 years of age are HIV seropositive. Half of them will probably develop AIDS within ten years. About 40 percent of their children will be HIV infected and most will become ill and die within two years. Zambia is first coming to understand the severity of the problem, as the epidemic continues to take an especially heavy toll on the nation's leadership and middle class.

In Bangkok, Thailand, AIDS has begun to take hold. Nearly half of the 60,000 intravenous drug users, living in the slums near the canals, or klongs, of Bangkok have become recently HIV infected. The sex tours continue to bring in tourists from Japan, Singapore, Hong Kong, Europe, and elsewhere. Tens of thousands of bar girls and a thousand bar boys continue to engage in unprotected sex. Safer sex practices are only beginning to emerge in Thailand.

In the United States, AIDS is certainly as devastating as it has become in parts of Europe, Africa, Asia, and Latin America. Just when the lives of persons with hemophilia (about 20,000 in the United States) become appreciably enhanced with the development of factor VIII concentrate, allowing persons with hemophilia to lead healthier lives, along comes AIDS. Today, most persons with hemophilia in the United States are HIV–1 infected. Many have become gravely ill, many have died, many have infected their wives or sexual partners, some have infected their children. Persons with hemophilia, who have only recently lifted the stigma of having a poorly understood disease associated by the public in the past with royal inbreeding and pejoratively called the "bleeder's disease," are now finding themselves labeled with an even more stigmatized disease, AIDS, which is associated in the public consciousness with immorality, "promiscuity," drug addiction, and "perversion." One major hemophilia organization in the United States in 1987 lost a $25,000 annual grant from a corporate sponsor, because the corporation wished to be no longer associated with helping people with hemophilia since they were identified by the public as persons at risk for AIDS. Also, many of the hemophilia organization's group activities for families have been eroded with a substantial loss in participation by families who feel uncomfortable about their HIV seropositive status.

Just when gay and bisexual men (estimated by some with a population of between six and ten million in the United States) begin to emerge out of a profound state of political and interpersonal oppression, AIDS strikes. By the early 1980s, a substantial proportion of American heterosexuals stopped viewing homosexuals as sinners, or criminals, or as mentally ill. Many began to first view the gay community as a viable sociocultural alternative, functioning as if it were a cohesive ethnic group within a pluralistic society. Johnny Carson, a popular American television personality and comedian, began to substitute his occasional anti-gay humor for jokes directed against such homophobic leaders as Anita Bryant and the Reverend Jerry Falwell.

The gay community established a unique identity through the proliferation of gay bars, gay bath houses, gay newspapers, gay magazines, gay radio and cable television programming, gay doctors, gay dentists, gay lawyers, gay hotels, and a multiplicity of gay social and political organizations. *Gayellow Pages,* a directory of gay businesses and services in the United States, lists over 10,000 entries.

It is likely that about 15 to 20 percent of all gay and bisexual men in the United States are HIV–1 seropositive (between an estimated 0.9 million and 2.0 million persons). Unless a cure is somehow found, nearly all of these men may become dependent on antiviral and immunosupportive drug therapy in order to attempt to prevent the onset of AIDS-related symptoms during the next two decades.

AIDS has already had a profound effect on gay American culture. The number of gay bars and bath houses have substantially decreased in most large American cities, while new services, such as gay telephone party lines and all-male video tapes, have flourished. Gay visibility has declined in response to the new public perception and scorn of homosexuals as "diseased," and in response to the rise in violent attacks and verbal abuse (usually by male teenagers) against gay men and those whom are perceived to be gay.

Most American gay men practice safer sex techniques and have fewer partners, or have become monogamous. Many have become celibate out of fear of being infected, or (among those who know they are HIV seropositive) fear of infecting others. Some fatalistic or intractable gay men have not changed their sexual behavior at all.

There is considerable variability among gay men as to what exactly is safer sex. Receptive oral sex without a condom, active oral sex without a condom but without swallowing semen or preejaculatory fluid, and rectal insertion of one or more fingers without a condom are defined by some gay men as unsafe and by others as safer sex. Several years after AIDS was first reported in the medical literature, researchers have not yet provided gay and bisexual men with all the data necessary to completely protect themselves during sex. Just when the American gay community builds an alternative culture within a culture, accepting within itself that "gay is good," and rejecting a sense of personal shame for group pride, AIDS emerges.

Just when the tens of millions of sexually active heterosexual American men and women succeed in eradicating the vestiges of Victorian morality to forge a new sexual revolution which is committed to sexual freedom, equality between the sexes, the primacy of the rights of the individuals, and a sex-positive social environment, along comes AIDS. And just when tens of thousands of intravenous drug users (IVDUs) throughout the United States succeed with methadone and other treatment programs in ridding themselves of this addiction, and are successful in beginning a new career, to marry, and to build a family, once again, along comes AIDS, years later after their addiction has become a nightmarish memory, and years after their silent infection begins through shared needles of HIV. The spouse in some cases may not have known their partner was an IVDU, only to learn this when their partner develops AIDS and the spouse and often the children test HIV seropositive.

AIDS is a dreadful disease. But almost as bad as the disease itself, has been the public reaction to it. The early days when physicians and nurses dared approach a person with AIDS (PWA) only if fully gowned, masked, and gloved are fortunately gone in nearly all North American hospitals. More and more ambulance services and funeral homes have become equipped to handle PWAs. There is little public outcry heard today to keep children with HIV infection out of schools. But in many other areas—in housing, in employment, in insurance, in many health services—PWAs are finding themselves the continuing objects of AIDS-related discrimination.

Fear, bigotry, and misinformation are the key sources of AIDS-related discrimination on virtually every level of social interaction. In some cases, government officials, politicians, and civic leaders have mobilized widespread fear, bigotry, and misinformation to politicize the disease and promote their own restrictive agenda in the United States.

In West Virginia, a municipal swimming pool was closed down after it was discovered that an HIV-infected person had swam in the pool. In Acadia, Florida, the house belonging to a family that included three HIV seropositive children with hemophilia was burned to the ground. In New York City, a home designated to house "border babies" (homeless infants) was firebombed when it was discovered that some of the infants would have AIDS.

Again in New York City, a community-based AIDS service and educational organization formed to help PWAs, educate the public about the disease, and to fight against AIDS-related discrimination (The AIDS Center of Queens County), found itself the target when a local politician and neighborhood block association demanded its relocation out of their area. They sustained a rock through their window, a gun shot through their front door, damage to their employees' cars, and threats of physical violence, firebombing, and mass demonstrations. The matter resolved itself when the New York State Department of Health worked out a solution that resulted in the dissolution of the organization's leadership and the relocation of the AIDS center out of the neighborhood. And in Chicago, inadequate AIDS funding had severely polarized the gay and black communities during the late 1980s. Moreover, throughout the world AIDS has been used as an excuse to promote sexually restrictive agendas that condemn premarital sex, extramarital sex, homosexuality, and prostitution even in areas where the prevailing norms had previously been less restrictive.

The AIDS crisis has brought out the worst in some people, but then the best in others. Over two thousand persons, mostly gay men, are currently volunteering to serve as "buddies" to help PWAs in their homes at the Gay Men's Health Crisis (GMHC), the world's largest AIDS service delivery and educational organization located in New York City. Hundreds of additional volunteers have been referred by GMHC to other AIDS community-based organizations during the late 1980s.

Though a relentless and tragic human disaster, the advent of AIDS has also led to greater safeguards taken by surgeons, dentists, and other health professionals in avoiding not only HIV infection, but also hepatitis B and other pathogens. It has forced us not only to screen our blood supply for HIV, but to begin a program against HTLV–1—a carcinogenic retrovirus.

AIDS has also forced us to look much more critically at the inadequacies of our health care system in the United States: at our poorly funded and failing municipal hospitals, at the lack of health insurance among tens of millions of Americans and the need for national health insurance, and at the early lethargy on the part of the Food and Drug Administration in releasing experimental antiretroviral drugs to PWAs on a compassionate basis. It has also caused us to look at America's inadequate commitment to funding health and medical needs in the developing world.

Perhaps we stand not at the precipice of global chaos and disaster, but at the gateway for a world that is concerned about the health needs of all its population, for a planet that will rectify its serious deficiencies in health care delivery, for a world where the rights of persons with AIDS take precedence over the stigma of AIDS. In the United States, AIDS has crystallized what is wrong with the health care system. We need to utilize that clarity to build an equitable and efficient health care system for all. We need to utilize the inadequacies existing within our society that have been illuminated by our reaction to AIDS, in order to work toward promoting much needed social and cultural change.

A culture, in a specific sense, is a particular way of life. But, in a broad sense, *Culture* is the intricate process by humans of sharing language, utilizing symbols, and organizing and giving meaning to behavior. Culture includes family organization, politics, law, religion, art, music, language, health care, magic, sexual behavior, and any other capability acquired by humans within a social setting. It is learned, shared behavior passed intergenerationally. A cultural understanding focuses not only upon *what* humans do, nor only upon *how* we do it, but upon *why* we do it. An analysis of cultural change is not merely interested in what has changed and how it has changed, but why it has changed. Anthropologists have learned through cross-cultural research that human behavior is highly explainable, and to that extent (within a range) largely predictable. AIDS can be understood as a cultural phenomenon, and social patterning of the global pandemic can be explained and its direction generally predicted.

We also know that AIDS is a preventable disease and culture-specific interventions can substantially reduce the future spread of AIDS throughout the world. On a global level, about ten million persons are HIV infected, about half of them in Africa. Social science research on AIDS in the Third World attempts to understand the pattern of social epidemiologic spread and to assess the social services needs of persons with AIDS and their families and/or loved ones. It also attempts to understand the cultural processes that are essential to developing culture-specific AIDS education campaigns and risk reduction workshops. People need more than culturally appropriate knowledge about AIDS; they need to have effective risk reduction workshops that utilize role-playing techniques to gain the social skills to practice safer sex and to eliminate needle-sharing risk. Knowledge is rarely sufficient to change people's learned behavior.

This volume, written almost entirely by anthropologists united in the struggle against AIDS, looks at the meaning of AIDS in Rwanda (central Africa), how one Haitian village handles AIDS in their midst, possible cofactors in HIV transmission, social service needs of gay men with AIDS in New York City, how psychological factors influence adjustment among HIV-infected gay men in Houston, social behavior of female prostitutes in London, the social effects of AIDS on minority women, the role of AIDS-related stigma in the press, the relationship between language and AIDS, and other AIDS-related areas. The chapters were written specifically for this volume. It is the hope of the editor that this book will considerably broaden the way the reader thinks about AIDS and how it is changing our lives as it re-directs human experience.

# Chapter Two

## AIDS in Cultural, Historic, and Epidemiologic Context

### S. C. McCombie

## INTRODUCTION

We shall never return to the demonic and miasmatic theories of the past, and the practical application of the principles developed by a series of clear thinkers and brilliant investigators—from Fracastorius to Chapin—has forever banished from the earth the major plagues and pestilences of the past. (Winslow, 1943:380)

All human societies, past and present, have suffered from infectious diseases. The belief systems of many traditional societies contain elements that are compatible with a notion of contagion. Although the idea of contagion is very ancient, the germ theory of disease did not gain acceptance in Western medical theory until the bacteriological work of Louis Pasteur and Robert Koch in the late nineteenth century. Following their discoveries, an explosion in knowledge regarding the etiological agents and modes of transmission of a large number of human diseases occurred. The development and widespread use of vaccines, antibiotics, and insecticides gave Western society a sense of control and victory over nature, and led to great optimism about the potential for eliminating infectious disease.

In 1980, when the World Health Organization declared that smallpox had been eradicated, few physicians or scientists would have believed that a new and virulent infectious agent was beginning to spread throughout the world. The success of the smallpox eradication program had reinforced the notion that mortality from infectious disease was a thing of the past. Attention had already begun to focus on "non-infectious" disease, the chronic and degenerative diseases that had emerged as the leading causes of death in developed countries. Diet, life-style, and environmental factors were considered to be the important causes of these conditions, and prevention efforts focused on altering the related behaviors. The view that the battle against infectious disease had been won was widespread, but not universal.

Some physicians share the widely held view that the era of discovery of new human pathogens is over, an indictment not applicable to the infectious disease specialist. We are overwhelmed with newly recognized clinical entities, produced by agents both old and new. (Weller, 1980:458)

Those who were familiar with the properties of infectious disease agents and their capacity for evolving were less optimistic about their imminent disappearance (Mims, 1980). In addition, infectious agents were beginning to be recognized as the causes of some of the chronic and degenerative diseases. Wolf (1980:100) suggested that the term "degenerative" was merely a mask for current ignorance and stated,

During the last 30 years, degeneration and abiotrophy have failed us because, one by one, diseases which have been classified as degenerative dementias, hereditary abiotrophies, or metabolic remote effects of cancer have been revealed as infectious, due to transmissible agents that may be isolated and characterized. (Wolf, 1980:251)

Several separate lines of study were leading researchers in this direction. One was the discovery of slow viruses (now termed prions) as the etiological agents in human neurological diseases such as kuru (Gajdusek et al., 1966) and Creutzfeldt-Jakob disease (Gibbs et al., 1968). Associations between human tumors and viruses had been documented as early as 1965 (Epstein et al., 1965). Another line of study was the long-standing research regarding retroviruses. A retrovirus had been identified as the cause of chicken sarcoma as early as 1910 (Gilden and McAllister, 1982:22). Over the next several decades retroviruses were discovered to be the cause of leukemias, lymphomas, and sarcomas in a large number of animal species (Gross, 1970) and suspicions that viruses would also be linked to human malignancies became increasingly common (Vianna, 1975; Francis and Essex, 1978; Gross, 1978, 1980).

The search for a human retrovirus had persisted for half a century (Blattner, 1987:1795). These efforts proved successful in the early 1980s when the retrovirus now termed human T-cell leukemia virus type I (HTLV-I) was documented to be the cause of adult T-cell leukemia (Poiesz et al., 1980, 1981; Popovic et al., 1983). However, the significance of these events was not widely appreciated, and they had little impact on the prevailing philosophies in medicine and public health.

## THE DISCOVERY OF AIDS

"It is not clear if or how the clustering of Kaposi's sarcoma, pneumocystis, and other serious disease in homosexual men is related" (Centers for Disease

Control, 1981b:307). In June 1981 the *Morbidity and Mortality Weekly Report* reported on 5 cases of *Pneumocystis carinii* pneumonia (PCP) in previously healthy gay men from Los Angeles (Centers for Disease Control, 1981a). This was the first indication of immune deficiency in this population. Pneumocystis carinii is an opportunistic parasite that normally causes disease only in individuals whose immune systems are suppressed due to cancer, leukemia, lymphoma, immuno-suppressive drugs or extreme malnutrition. Within a month, a second report was published in the *Morbidity and Mortality Weekly Report* describing the occurrence of Kaposi's sarcoma (KS) in 20 gay men from New York and 6 from Los Angeles (Centers for Disease Control, 1981b). At that time, KS was a rare malignancy in the United States, and was almost totally confined to elderly men of Mediterranean descent. KS was also known to be associated with immunosuppression. The appearance of these two diseases in previously healthy young men suggested a common underlying immunodeficiency that was related in some way to the life-style of gay men. News of the syndrome reached the general public through the mass media in late 1981 with headlines such as, "Diseases that Plague Gays" (Clark and Gosnell, 1981:51). Early reports characterized the syndrome as mysterious and deadly (Opportunistic diseases, 1981:68).

Over the next year, the number of reported cases continued to grow, and by the end of 1982 the syndrome had been reported in intravenous drug users, hemophiliacs, Haitians, blood transfusion recipients, and infants. Many of these reports were based on retrospective review. The term "AIDS" came into wide-spread use in late 1982. To the media and the public, the temporal sequence of reported cases was seen as equivalent to the temporal sequence of case occurrence, and the view that AIDS was "spreading from" gay men to other groups became prevalent. The initial association of the syndrome with what many in society considered a deviant life-style had a profound impact on the way in which researchers, the media, and the public responded to the new disease.

Early hypotheses regarding the etiology of AIDS focused on a number of factors. Some theorized that the act of anal intercourse itself resulted in immunosuppression (Richards et al., 1984). The use of amyl and butyl nitrates (poppers) was also suspected to have a role in causing the syndrome. Although many suspected that a transmissible agent was the cause, this hypothesis did not receive widespread official support, even after reports of clusters of cases among sexual partners (Centers for Disease Control, 1982:307). After the syndrome was reported in hemophiliacs and other recipients of blood products, the transmissible agent hypothesis became the focus of most serious consideration.

## THE DISCOVERY AND CHARACTERIZATION
## OF HIV AND RELATED ILLNESS

"[T]here will be a survival advantage to a virus strain if it can mutate to a new type not blocked by antibody against the old" (Burnet, 1962:27). By 1984, one laboratory in France and two in the United States had isolated retroviruses from persons who had AIDS or were at high risk for the disease (Barre-Sinoussi et al., 1983; Popovic et al., 1984; Levy et al., 1984). Three separate names came into use: lymphadenopathy-associated virus (LAV), human T-cell leukemia/lymphotropic virus, type III (HTLV-III) and AIDS-associated retrovirus (ARV). Over the next two years clinical and serological research led to general agreement that these isolates represented variants of a single type of retrovirus which was the probable cause of AIDS. During this time controversy developed over which group deserved credit for the discovery, and what the appropriate nomenclature should be. In 1986, the International Committee on Taxonomy of Viruses recommended the designation: human immunodeficiency virus (HIV).

In a relatively short time period, a great deal of knowledge was accumulated regarding the biology, pathogenesis, and natural history of infection with HIV. Application of serological testing revealed a wide range of clinical manisfestations associated with HIV, including asymptomatic carriage for several years, nonspecific symptoms (often called AIDS-related complex) such as fever, diarrhea, weight loss, and generalized lymphadenopathy-increased susceptibility to certain opportunistic pathogens, increased severity of infection with certain conventional pathogens, development of malignancies including KS, primary lymphoma of the brain, other non-Hodgkin's lymphomas, and progressive encephalopathy (HIV dementia).

As the spectrum of illness associated with HIV expanded, the utility of the surveillance definition of AIDS used by the Centers for Disease Control in collecting case reports came under question. The case definition, which had undergone minor revisions and additions between 1982 and 1986, was designed to count only documented infections or malignancies that indicated severe immunodeficiency and occurred in the absence of known causes of reduced resistance. For each indicator disease, there were specific criteria for establishing a definitive diagnosis. Invasive procedures such as bronchoscopy or biopsy, and sophisticated laboratory analysis were often needed to establish that a patient had "CDC-defined" AIDS. If the specified tests were not done or were negative, the patient was not counted as an official AIDS case. In addition, morbidity and mortality due to AIDS-related complex, wasting syndrome, and encephalopathy were not included. Concern developed that a significant amount of HIV-related disease was being overlooked. In September 1987, a new surveillance definition with extensive changes was published (Centers for Disease Control, 1987) in an attempt to incorporate a broader range of HIV-related disease. Presumptive as well as definitive criteria for the diagnosis of opportunistic infections were listed, and HIV wasting syndrome and HIV dementia were added. A number of new infections and malignancies were added. Laboratory evidence of HIV infection (antibody testing, viral culture, or antigen detection) was also required in most of the cases.

An examination of the clinical spectrum of HIV-related disease and the changes in criteria for CDC-defined AIDS reveals a conceptual paradox for epidemiologists that has resulted from the discovery of AIDS and of HIV. "AIDS" is neither a disease nor a syndrome as traditionally defined. To have "AIDS," one must have some other disease, such as *Pneumocystis carinii* pneumonia or Kaposi's sarcoma. A person with "AIDS" may have both PCP and KS, as well as some other indicator disease, such as a herpes lesion that is progressive and fails to heal after four weeks. But a person with HIV infection who becomes ill and dies does not have "AIDS" unless evidence for one of these or a number of other conditions is found. Thus, "AIDS" is defined in relationship to other known diseases. The statements "He has AIDS because he has PCP" and "He has PCP because he has AIDS" are both correct. The first describes the diagnosis of AIDS based on evidence for an opportunistic infection, the second describes the development of an opportunistic infection as a result of severe immunodeficiency.

The conceptual paradox created by defining a disease or syndrome in relationship to other diseases has a number of implications for the classification of disease and for the analysis of morbidity and mortality data. AIDS provides a framework for illustrating the limitations of the current system for classifying cause of death. The rules for coding cause of death instruct the coder to choose the underlying condition that led to death (U.S. Dept. of Health and Human Services, 1987). If a person who has leukemia develops PCP, the primary cause of death will be counted as leukemia, and not PCP. Similarly, a person who is hospitalized after an accident and dies as a result of a nosocomial infection acquired in the hospital will most likely be listed as dying from an accident, and not an infection. Apparent changes in patterns of mortality can sometimes be due to changes in emphasis or diagnosis by mortality coders or physicians who prepare death certificates (Sorlie and Gold, 1987).

These limitations in classifying cause of death are likely to be magnified by AIDS as currently defined. Deaths due to conditions such as non-Hodgkin's lymphoma, disseminated coccidioidomycosis, or abdominal tuberculosis may now be reported as AIDS deaths if the person is HIV positive. In some cases, a person may meet the criteria for AIDS although HIV infection was acquired recently and had no impact on the disease process leading to death. As more persons become infected with the virus and are identified by antibody testing, more deaths may be attributed to AIDS and fewer to other diseases. At the same time, AIDS deaths are underrepresented when pneumonia and other conditions are recorded on death certificates without reference to HIV. Lack of standardization in the preparation and coding of death certificates is already a significant problem. In order to characterize the impact of HIV and other diseases more adequately, researchers may be forced into greater reliance on analyses of multiple causes of death.

The recognition of AIDS and discovery of HIV represent events that could not have occurred without the advances in virology and immunology that preceded them. In linking two separate disease syndromes (PCP and KS) under a common syndrome, epidemiologists created a conceptual paradox at the same time they removed one of the major obstacles that had prevented viruses from being established as the cause of human chronic diseases. In this instance, the one agent/one disease requirement was abandoned, and the actual complexity of disease etiology was exposed to study.

## THE IMPLICATIONS OF HIV
## FOR EVOLUTIONARY BIOLOGY

"Clearly such rapid evolution of RNA viruses could pose challenges to immune systems despite their own diversity" (Holland et al., 1982:1583). Because of the existing knowledge of the genetic organization of retroviruses and availability of new technologies for gene cloning and DNA sequencing, understanding of the molecular biology of HIV has proceeded rapidly, and in some ways exceeds that of most other known human viruses. Most researchers have classified HIV with the lentiviruses, cytopathic retroviruses that cause progressive illness in sheep (visna virus) and horses (equine infectious anemia virus). HIV is similar to the human T-cell leukemia viruses (HTLV-I and HTLV-II) in that its major target cells are OKT4 lymphocytes (Rabson and Martin, 1985:478).

HIV isolates show a considerable amount of genetic heterogeneity, particularly in the envelope (env) gene (Alizon et al., 1986:63). Considerable differences have been found in isolates from different geographic areas as well as isolates from the same individual at different points in time (Hahn et al., 1986:1548). This heterogeneity has been proposed to occur as a result of immune selection and may be one of the mechanisms by which HIV maintains persistent infection in a single host. These findings have led to skepticism about the potential for prevention of AIDS by vaccination (Ho et al., 1987:283) and suggests that HIV represents an example of micro-level evolutionary adaptation. To complicate matters further, additional retroviruses (LAV-II, HTLV-IV) have been isolated in Africa (Clavel et al., 1986; Kanki et al., 1986). These strains are genetically distinct from HIV-I, and unlike any other known human virus. LAV-II has been associated with an AIDS-like disease (Clavel et al., 1986). Most of these new isolates are now being classified as strains of HIV-II.

The evolutionary implications of RNA viruses were beginning to be explored prior to the discovery of HIV-I. Because retroviruses possess reverse transciptase and are consequently transcribed into DNA, they have the potential to play an important role in shaping the genome of their hosts. RNA viruses have extremely high rates of mutation, because they lack the proofreading enzymes of DNA (Holland et al., 1982:1577). In recent years a number of new discoveries have occurred in molecular genetics, many of which were unexpected and have resulted in significant challenges to traditional evolutionary theory. The properties of introns, exons, repetitive DNA, pseudogenes and gene transfer have just begun to be extensively studied.

It has been suggested that retroviruses may be a mechanism by which genes are transferred to different chromosomes (Leder et al., 1981:198; Baltimore,

1985). The role of viruses in gene transfer between hosts and possibly between species has also been considered (Gilden and McAllister, 1982:252; Nei, 1987:121). Retroviruses themselves can undergo recombination and gene transfer, and two viruses may appear more closely related than they actually are because of apparent homologies produced by such events (Chiu et al., 1984:364).

Because of the serious public health implications of AIDS, a great deal of attention and research is now being directed at HIV-I and related viruses. The information being gathered has obvious implications for virology, immunology, and oncology. Understanding of HIV-I will also have implications for our understanding of molecular evolution. The discovery of the genetic variability and unusual features of HIV-I has brought viruses again to the attention of evolutionary biologists. The role of these ubiquitous and transmissible packets of genetic material in evolution can no longer be overlooked.

## THE ORIGIN OF HIV-I

"There is, therefore a serious danger that viruses from such closely related groups as the simian primates could show an altered pathogenesis in man, of which malignancy could be a feature" (Fiennes, 1967:144). A desire to understand the origin of things derives from a basic human curiosity and underlies much of anthropological research and theory. Questions related to origin characterize a substantial portion of other scientific endeavors as well. In the case of most infectious diseases, hypotheses regarding their origin are speculative and untestable.

Like HIV-I, the viruses that cause measles and smallpox are highly species specific, and rarely infect or cause disease in other animals. Yet disease theorists have usually hypothesized an animal origin for measles and smallpox. The existence of closely related viruses in domestic animals is used as evidence (Cockburn, 1971:51). This type of evidence is equally supportive of the hypothesis that the animals in question acquired their diseases from contact with humans. However, Western scientists try to find the cause of disease in "nature" rather than in humans (McCombie, 1985:26).

For the layperson, when the topic is an infectious agent that produces human suffering and death, the question of origin becomes confused with the idea of responsibility. In many societies, epidemics are viewed as unnatural events brought on by various taboo violations. Even in modern Western cultures, victim blaming and viewing disease as punishment from God are frequent. Throughout history, disease has often been blamed on "outsiders," as defined by race, ethnicity, religion, or nationality.[1] In Western cultural concepts, disease is considered unnatural, and the genesis of disease is best placed as far from "people like us" as possible. "Outsiders" may be humans who are different, or better yet, some other animal species.

Speculation concerning the origin of AIDS provides a modern example of these tendencies. An elaborate evolutionary scenario involving green monkeys,

Africans, Haitians, and vacationing American homosexuals has been constructed. For various political and economic reasons, aspects of this scenario have become the subject of a bitter controversy (Norman, 1985:1140). In the form it has taken in the lay press, this scenario has all of the characteristics of a "just so" story. As related in the December 1985 issue of *Discover*, the progenitor of HIV-I is found in the African green monkey. People in Central Africa who ate or were bitten by the monkeys acquired the virus, which was then transmitted to Haitians visiting Zaire. In Haiti, vacationing American homosexuals acquired the infection, and brought it back to New York (Langone, 1985:32–33).

The evidence for this hypothesized chain of events is fragmentary, and has sometimes been contradicted by subsequent research. Some have questioned the accuracy of the testing that showed the presence of HIV-I antibody in Central Africa prior to 1979 (Biggar, 1986:80). A number of authors have suggested that AIDS, while spreading rapidly, is a new disease in most parts of Africa, and began to appear at roughly the same time it did in the United States (Van de Perre et al., 1984:68; Clumeck et al., 1984:497; Biggar, 1986; Feldman, 1986).

Regardless of whether HIV-I existed in Africa before appearing in other parts of the world, the impact of this assertion has already occurred. For many of the people who have been exposed to the media reports, it has become a fact. Cultural myths die hard, and the association of AIDS with Africa has become as much a part of American cultural attitudes toward the disease as its association with homosexuality.

The green monkey link to AIDS has recently been discredited. DNA sequencing of both viruses has shown that the monkey retrovirus (simian immunodeficiency virus—SIV)[2] shares less than half of its nucleotides with HIV-I, making it unlikely that SIV is a recent progenitor of HIV (Guo et al., 1987:183). However, the idea of a monkey progenitor, once proposed, becomes as difficult to eradicate as a retrovirus. In *Nature* the consensus that the SIV is not the recent ancestor of HIV-I was presented. The author suggested that the progenitor of HIV-I may be a monkey virus that has yet to be found (Newmark, 1987:458). Apparently, myths die hard among scientists as well.

## CONTROVERSIES SURROUNDING SEXUAL TRANSMISSION OF HIV

The level of alarm over this pandemic is substantial and appropriate. We should not raise that level with conjecture about female-to-male transmission, but should embrace the null hypothesis until it is wrested from us by valid data. We may hope that the null hypothesis will not be rejected. (Polk, 1985:3178)

Cultural attitudes have also had an impact on the accumulation and dissemination of information regarding transmission of HIV. A great deal of resistance to the idea of heterosexual transmission emerged early in the pandemic, even in the face of strong evidence. Common sense should tell one that a virus ignores the sex of its potential host. Yet some have received the claims of heterosexual transmission with astonishment, skepticism, and outright denial.

The occurrence of AIDS in heterosexual partners of cases was reported in 1982 (Masur et al., 1982) but received little attention. For some the fact that AIDS in Africa appeared to be primarily a heterosexually transmitted disease (Van de Perre et al., 1984:62; Clumeck et al., 1985:2599) was evidence that the virus could be transmitted bidirectionally through vaginal intercourse, although perhaps with less efficiency than by anal intercourse. For others, the discrepancy between the epidemiology of AIDS in Africa and the United States was interpreted in a number of other ways. The idea that the AIDS virus in Africa or that the African people themselves were "different" was proposed. An extreme view along these lines is seen in statements such as "it is impossible to generalize from Africa about the ways in which AIDS may spread in the west" (Fitzpatrick and Milligan, 1987:7). Insect transmission, use of contaminated needles for the treatment of sexually transmitted disease (Kreiss et al., 1986:417; Seale, 1985:71), and unreported homosexuality (Fitzpatrick and Milligan, 1987:7) have been among the explanations proposed to account for the equal sex distribution of cases in Africa.

The occurrence of female-to-male transmission was even more difficult for some to accept than the possibility for male-to-female transmission. Some went to extraordinary lengths to explain away cases of female-to-male transmission. " . . . it is possible that the disease was in fact acquired from infected sperm of a prior customer of the prostitute that remained alive in the vaginal canal—a sort of quasi-homosexual contact" (Kant, 1985:1901).

The idea that male-to-female transmission could occur but that female-to-male transmission was physically impossible was common during the period beginning in 1985 when heterosexual transmission began to be discussed widely. It is interesting and perhaps not simply coincidental that this viewpoint fits nicely with the double standard of sexuality in American culture. For those who believed in unidirectional transmission, a man who had sex with many women could not be at risk, but a woman who had sex with many men would be at risk. Thus, "promiscuity" would be safe for men but not for women. The question then becomes, does the transmission of this virus accidentally conform to a cultural ideal, or has the cultural ideal influenced both the scientific and lay interpretation of the evidence?

The isolation of virus in cervical secretions (Vogt et al., 1986) and epidemiologic evidence for female-to-male transmission (Fischl et al., 1987) has set the issue to rest for some. For many the debate goes on, although modified into concerns regarding the relative efficiency of heterosexual transmission. The amount of resources devoted to understanding the magnitude of risk of HIV transmission through various types of sexual contact is unprecedented when compared to epidemiologic research of other infectious diseases.

## CONTAGION IN CULTURAL AND HISTORICAL PERSPECTIVE

We need to stop the spread of AIDS. I feel it's a judgement from God, and we need to stop it any way we can.

I'm not convinced that if I walk into a restaurant I'm not going to walk out with AIDS or walk out with the virus or something like that. These days I'm walking around Tucson, breathing the air, I'm liable to get something. (Statements made at a public hearing regarding an ordinance to regulate adult amusement establishments. Pima County, Arizona, July 28, 1987.)

The concept of contagion has a long history in Western society. A number of diseases were recognized as contagious long before the official acceptance of the germ theory in the late nineteenth century, including plague, smallpox, measles, leprosy, tuberculosis, and scabies. During periods in history when medical writers downplayed contagion and stressed humoral and miasmatic explanations of epidemics, a belief in contagion was sometimes prevalent among laymen, and could be seen in the writings of poets and historians (Winslow, 1943:81–85). In 1910, Charles Chapin described the over-isolation of the sick, and the tendency of the American public to exaggerate the role of airborne transmission in spreading infection (Chapin, 1910).

A tendency to overemphasize the transmissibility of a disease and the role of inanimate objects in spreading infection is prominent in contemporary American society. As recently as 1947, hepatitis was considered to be transmitted by a respiratory route (Francis, 1947:654). This belief persists among many laypersons and some medical personnel and is used as a justification for isolation and exclusion of affected individuals from routine daily activities (McCombie, 1986).

Confusion about the mode of transmission of specific infectious diseases has occurred throughout history and has resulted in inappropriate control measures. The isolation of persons with leprosy, a disease now known to be of low infectivity, was practiced for centuries. Health officials recommended the isolation of persons with polio and their household contacts even after it was known that there were hundreds of asymptomatic infections for every case of paralytic disease (Payne, 1955:388). The widely held idea that venereal diseases such as syphilis were easily transmitted by drinking cups, shared personal items, and food handlers can be traced to the statements of the very physicians who specialized in the treatment of syphilis (Pusey, 1915:119). Requirements that domestic workers and food handlers be tested for venereal diseases reinforced these notions, although the health officials who supported them saw their function primarily as case finding (Brandt, 1985:157).

Public fear about acquiring AIDS through various sorts of casual contact has been an important aspect of the cultural response to the disease at all stages of the epidemic. The resulting attempts at discrimination against people with AIDS or people considered to be at high risk for AIDS have become so widely known that almost every medical or public health protocol mentions the phenomenon. In some cases, features of the policies are specifically geared toward dealing with these issues. The following quote illustrates some of the public responses that have made it impossible to deal with AIDS without considering discrimination and disclosure issues.

Although our understanding of the disease has been progressing rapidly, the new knowledge has often produced more public concern than relief. The identification of the etiologic agent as a virus—although of critical scientific importance—did little to quell the fears of either the medical community or the general population.

The belief that the AIDS virus can be transmitted by casual contact has produced numerous political, legal and ethical dilemmas. Responses have been varied, including calls for quarantine, mass screening of all potentially infected persons, expulsion from military service of all antibody positive personnel, and exclusion of infected children from schools. In some cases refusal to care for AIDS patients has been condoned. (Sande, 1986:380)

In the bitter debate that has come to surround these issues, a frequent topic concerns the extent of scientific knowledge accumulated regarding transmission of HIV. A concern often voiced by those who favor isolation and exclusion is, "We just don't know enough about this virus. It's too new." The impact of the mass media is considerable. Press coverage of a handful of cases of transmission to health care workers is extensive and sensational, but the much larger number of studies showing lack of transmission do not receive media attention. In some cases, physicians and other medical professionals have shared and reinforced the public's concerns. Elford (1987:547) notes that anxiety about HIV transmission through glasses or cutlery never completely disappeared among a group of medical students in spite of intensive education. Statements from physicians such as "the risk, however minimal, is too great" (physician from Arcadia, Florida, quoted in O'Brien, 1987:34) add to the public's fears and have convinced some that public officials are being less than honest about HIV transmission.

This controversy may be viewed as a clash of two cultures. An epidemiologist's understanding of the transmission of infectious disease is much different from a layperson's, and is characterized by the classification of disease agents into specific categories such as fecal, oral, respiratory, vector borne, and sexually transmitted. For many laypersons, disease is classified in a much more undifferentiated way, that is, contagious, very contagious, and not contagious. Thus, once AIDS becomes glossed as "contagious" it may be spread in all sorts of ways, even if it is understood to be "not very contagious."

The connection of the term "virus" to AIDS may also impute a certain association with "contagiousness." A quote from a mental health practitioner illustrates this. "When experts say that AIDS is not transmitted by casual contact, what do they mean? Is it transmitted like other viruses?" (Conant, 1986:25, emphasis added). The term "virus," which signifies a specific type of disease agent to an epidemiologist, means something entirely different to the lay public and some in the medical profession, who use the term to describe febrile illnesses that seem to "go around" (McCombie, 1987).

Some cite the high fatality rate as an explanation for excessive concern and over-isolation. But hysteria and over-isolation have also occurred with herpes ("Confusion," 1984:73; "Herpes," 1984:1). In addition, successful lawsuits in favor of those who acquired herpes from a sex partner have been adjudicated (Hernandez, 1986; Goode, 1987:66) and have set the stage for similar types of litigation concerning AIDS.

## CONTROVERSIES REGARDING CONTROL MEASURES: THE EXAMPLE OF SYPHILIS

It is strictly a disease of man; and it is one of the most important diseases that afflict him. It has the tragic human interest of being hereditary—hereditary as no other important disease is; a disease that may pass as such from parent to child. Its manifestations are so varied that, in the words of Johnathan Hutchinson, "It is an epitome of pathology," and its study is one of the interests of every branch of medicine. It is surely the most difficult of diseases from the point of view of sociology, for it is inextricably involved in the great unsolved problem of the relation of the sexes. And with all this, the history of syphilis is unique among the records of great diseases. For, unlike most diseases, it does not gradually emerge into the historical records of medicine and its characters become recognized, but appears on the stage of history with a dramatic suddenness in keeping with the tragic reputation it has made—as a great plague sweeping within a few years over the known world. (Pusey, 1915:9)

Complex legal, medical, and ethical issues have been raised in debates about the appropriate public health and legislative responses to AIDS. Various controversial measures have been proposed, including mandatory testing, quarantine, and criminal prosecution of those who "knowingly" transmit the virus. Opponents of such measures point out that such measures would drive persons at risk of infection away from sources of medical care and counseling and argue that coercion is ineffective in controlling sexual behavior and IV drug use. An increase in spread of infection could result. A large amount of literature has been published focusing on legal and ethical aspects of proposed control measures (Matthews and Neslund, 1987; Gostin and Curran, 1987; Gleason, 1986). The publication of a biweekly newsletter entitled *AIDS Policy and Law* attests to the widespread impact of these issues. The content of educational messages is also a subject of debate. Predictably, conservatives emphasize abstinence and monogamy as solutions, and deride any discussion of preventive measures such as condoms as a promotion of promiscuity.

On the surface, AIDS and the issues it has raised appear unique. To many involved in the present debates, AIDS is "different" than any other disease, and recent history provides little in the way of useful comparisons. But to the careful student of history, the issues raised regarding the control of AIDS are little more than a series of old arguments wearing new hats.

In 1915, the situation with syphilis was similar to that of AIDS today. The causal agent had been identified and a serological test (Wassermann reaction) had been developed to aid in the detection of the disease. The rapid and effective cure of penicillin did not yet exist. Treatment with the recently developed salvarsan was lengthy, toxic, and not always effective. Because patients could be rendered noninfectious and the late effects of syphilis prevented in many cases, there was a rational basis for case finding that does not yet exist for asymptomatic HIV infections.

Controversies similar to those regarding AIDS today abounded. Private physicians were often resistant to the idea of reporting syphilis cases to the health department, and argued that it would interfere with controlling the disease's spread (Brandt, 1985:42). Hospitals sometimes refused to admit patients with venereal diseases (Brandt, 1985:44–45).

During World War I, concern about the impact of venereal disease on the fighting forces became the justification for the arrest and quarantine of thousands of prostitutes and other women suspected of sexual promiscuity. Those found to be infected were held for treatment for an average of ten weeks in federally funded institutions (Brandt, 1985:89). Programs involving post-exposure chemical prophylaxis for soldiers were criticized for promoting illicit activities (Brandt, 1985:112).

In 1937, Thomas Parran, then Surgeon General of the United States, published *Shadow on the Land*, an attempt to educate the American people about the dangers of syphilis and to separate the moral issues from the medical issues to facilitate its control. A review of this volume adds credit to the idea that history repeats itself.

Parran recognized that the moral context of a disease had implications for its control. His discussion of public priorities and financial allocations for research work is reminiscent of some of the earliest complaints about the U.S. government's response to AIDS. "The lack of public knowledge about syphilis and the stigma that has been attached to it has resulted not only in a lack of public action, but also a dearth of research work" (Parran, 1937:284).

The limits of serological testing and dangers of false diagnosis were recognized in the statement " . . . no person should be labelled a syphilitic on the basis of a single laboratory test" (Parran, 1937:10). A discussion of the reason for the lack of premarital Wassermann testing in the Soviet Union echoes one of the modern day arguments against premarital HIV testing. "Most couples coming before the marriage clerk to have their union registered already have had sexual relations" (Parran, 1937:129).

Employment discrimination based on serological test results is another topic.

We ignored syphilis as a disease; considered it the result of sin; suppressed discussion and action. Now we are beginning to look for it at least, but when we find it most employers, whether in government or private industry, fail to employ. This defeats the very purpose of finding cases, which is to get them treated. It results in driving syphilis under cover. (Parran, 1937:201)

Parran favored widespread testing as a means of case finding. His goal was treatment, but he was not reluctant to point out incentives to private industry to find cases for him. "Life insurance companies might profitably make a Wassermann test in the medical examination of every applicant for a policy" (Parran, 1937:250).

A study of sexually transmitted disease reveals the complex interplay between cultural, political, and economic factors in a society's response to disease. The current debates surrounding serological testing for HIV and other proposed control measures for AIDS are taking place in a sociopolitical context in which the public health issues are interwoven with a number of other political and social issues. The inability of many legislators to separate the moral issues from the medical ones is creating obstacles to the dissemination of information aimed at facilitating behavior change. Reports of the growing numbers of cases fuel public panic and the result in increased support for coercive and punitive measures. AIDS is becoming increasingly politicized, and fear of the disease can be manipulated to justify various political and social agendas. The historical precedents for such events are recent and ominous. In *Mein Kampf*, Adolf Hitler wrote that syphilis was a symbol of degeneration and its persistence the result of a weak government.

In the case of syphilis especially the attitude of the state and public bodies was one of absolute capitulation. To combat this state of affairs something of far wider sweep should have been undertaken than was really done.

A determined decision to act in this manner will at the same time provide an obstacle against the further spread of venereal disease. It would then be a case, where necessary, of mercilessly isolating all incurables—perhaps a barbaric measure for those unfortunates—but a blessing for the present generation and for posterity. (Hitler, 1939:209, 216)

## CONCLUSION

"Infectious disease which antedated the emergence of humankind will last as long as humanity itself, and will surely remain, as it has been hitherto, one of the fundamental parameters and determinants of human history" (McNeill,

1976:291). AIDS has become a biological and social phenomenon of great importance. One thing that distinguishes the situation with AIDS today from prior epidemics is the mass media. Today information, whether right or wrong, is rapidly disseminated worldwide to millions of people. One researcher's theory or offhand comment today is transformed into a fact in tomorrow's headlines. Cultural beliefs and attitudes influence the scientific collection and interpretation of data, which are then viewed through the eyes of reporters. "News," by definition, focuses on things that have not happened before, are not widely known, and are perhaps extraordinary. In the public mind, the rare event may be perceived as commonplace. Misinterpretation and improper translation of technical terms adds to the confusion. Thus, for the average person, AIDS becomes a mysterious and deadly plague that is threatening society. Rarely heard are the facts that HIV is difficult to transmit and infection easy to prevent.

For an epidemiologist, AIDS is a new disease as well as a new way of thinking about disease. Its discovery and analysis represents great achievements in virology, oncology, and immunology. At the same time it is a tremendous public health threat and challenge to medical technology. Some believe that a promising cure or vaccine will eventually be found, and that current efforts to alter behavior as a means of controlling transmission will no longer be needed. The American cultural heritage with its emphasis on the triumph of science over nature creates and reinforces such beliefs. However, an understanding of the evolution of disease reveals this attitude to be shortsighted. The appearance of HIV is a lesson in the evolution of disease. It is likely that infectious agents will be found to be the ultimate cause of a great many diseases for which etiology is now unclear. These agents will continue to adapt and evolve and evade whatever technological innovations are thrown at them.

We are now moving onto a new world in which the natural history of disease is being rapidly distorted, and we must be always alert to look beyond the immediate effect of some new procedure to see what the logical outcome of its large scale use will be. Antimicrobial drugs, like measures to prevent the spread of infection or immunization procedures, are potent weapons, but to the biologist they are merely new factors introduced into the environment within which the microorganisms of infection must struggle to survive. We must never underestimate the potentialities of our enemies. (Burnet and White, 1972:185)

We may cure AIDS, but we won't eradicate infectious disease. At best, we can keep pace, reduce suffering, and begin to examine the process by which perceptions of disease engender prejudice, social disruption, and culture change.

## NOTES

1. In a survey of knowledge of AIDS in Rwanda, six out of twelve persons who responded to a question regarding the origin of AIDS said it came from America (Feldman et al., 1987:98).

2. Some isolates of SIV have been called simian t-lymphotropic virus type III (STLV-III).

## REFERENCES

Alizon, Marc; Wain-Hobson, Simon; Montagnier, Luc; and Pierre Sonigo. 1986. Genetic variability of the AIDS virus: Nucleotide sequence analysis of two isolates from African patients. *Cell* 46:63–74.

Baltimore, David. 1987. Retroviruses and retrotransposons: The role of reverse transcription in shaping the eukaryotic genome. *Cell* 40:481–2.

Barre-Sinoussi, F.; Chermann, J.C.; Rey, F.; et al. 1983. Isolation of a T-lymphotropic retrovirus from a patient at risk for acquired immunodeficiency syndrome (AIDS). *Science* 220:868–71.

Biggar, Robert J. 1986. The AIDS problem in Africa. *Lancet* January 11:79–82.

Blattner, William A. 1987. Human Retroviruses. In *Textbook of Pediatric Infectious Diseases*, pp. 1795–1809. R.D. Feigin and J.D. Cherry, eds. Philadelphia: W.B. Saunders Company.

Brandt, Allan M. 1985. *No magic bullet.* New York: Oxford University Press.

Burnet, F.M. 1962. Evolution made visible: Current changes in the pattern of virus disease. In *The Evolution of Living Organisms.* G.W. Leeper, ed. pp. 23–32. London: Cambridge University Press.

Burnet, F.M., and David O. White. 1972. *Natural history of infectious disease.* Cambridge: Cambridge University Press.

Centers for Disease Control. 1981a. Pneumocystis Pneumonia—Los Angeles. *Morbidity and Mortality Weekly Report* 30:250–52.

———. 1981b. Kaposi's Sarcoma and Pneumocystis pneumonia among homosexual men—New York City and California. *Morbidity and Mortality Weekly Report* 30:305–8.

———. 1982. A cluster of Kaposi's sarcoma and *Pneumocystis carinii* pneumonia among homosexual male residents of Los Angeles and Orange counties, California. *Morbidity and Mortality Weekly Report* 31:305–7.

———. 1987. Revision of the CDC surveillance definition for Acquired Immunodeficiency Syndrome. *Morbidity and Mortality Weekly Report Supplement.*

Chapin, Charles. 1910. *The sources and modes of infection.* New York: John Wiley and Sons.

Chiu, Ing-Ming; Callahan, Robert; Tronick, Steven R.; et al. 1984. Major Pol gene progenitors in the evolution of oncoviruses. *Science* 223:364–70.

Clark, Matt, and Mariana Gosnell. 1981. Diseases That Plague Gays. *Newsweek* 98:51–52. Dec. 21.

Clavel, Francois; Guetard, Denise; Brun-Vezinet, Francoise; et al. 1986. Isolation of a new human retrovirus from West African patients with AIDS. *Science* 233:343–46.

Clumeck, Nathan; Robert-Guroff, Marjorie; Van de Perre, Philippe; et al. 1985. Seroepidemiological studies of HTLV-III antibody prevalence among selected groups of heterosexual Africans. *Journal of the American Medical Association* 254:2599–2602.

Clumeck, Nathan; Sonnet, Jean; Taelman, Henri; et al. 1984. Acquired immunodeficiency syndrome in African patients. *New England Journal of Medicine* 310:492–97.

Cockburn, T. Aidan. 1971. Infectious diseases in ancient populations. *Current Anthropology* 12:45–62.

Conant, Marcus. 1986. Questions from mental health practitioners about AIDS. In *What to do about AIDS*, pp. 25–31. L. McKusick, ed. Berkeley: University of California Press.

Confusion over infant herpes. 1984. *Time* January 16:73.

Elford, Jonathan. 1987. Moral and social aspects of AIDS: A medical students' project. *Social Science and Medicine* 24:543–49.

Epstein, M.A.; Henle, G.; Achong, B.G. and Y.M. Barr. 1965. Morphological and Biological Studies on a Virus in Cultured Lymphoblasts from Burkitt's Lymphoma. *Journal of Experimental Medicine* 121:761–70.

Feldman, Douglas A. 1986. AIDS, Africa, and Anthropology. *Medical Anthropology Quarterly* 17:38–40.

Feldman, Douglas A.; Friedman, Samuel R.; and Don C. Des Jarlais. 1987. Public Awareness of AIDS in Rwanda. *Social Science and Medicine* 24:97–100.

Fiennes, Richard. 1967. *Zoonoses of Primates*. Ithaca: Cornell University Press.

Fischl, Margaret A.; Dickinson, Gordon M.; Scott, Gwendolyn B.; et al. 1987. Evaluation of heterosexual partners, children, and household contacts of adults with AIDS. *Journal of the American Medical Association* 257:640–44.

Fitzpatrick, Michael, and Don Milligan. 1987. *The Truth about the AIDS Panic*. London: Junius Publications Ltd.

Francis, Donald P., and M. Essex. 1978. Leukemia and Lymphomas: Infrequent Manisfestations of Common Viral Infections? *Journal of Infectious Disease* 38:916–23.

Francis, Thomas, Jr. 1947. Infectious hepatitis. In *Communicable Diseases*, pp. 652–63. F. H. Top, Sr. ed. St. Louis: The C. V. Mosby Company.

Gajdusek, D.C.; Gibbs, C.J., Jr.; and M. Alphers. 1966. Experimental transmission of a kuru-like syndrome to chimpanzees. *Nature* 209:794–96.

Gibbs, C.J., Jr.; Gajdusek, D.C.; Asher, D.M.; et al. 1968. Creutzfeldt-Jakob disease (spongiform encephalopathy); transmission to the chimpanzee. *Science* 161:388–89.

Gilden, Raymond V., and Robert M. McAllister. 1982. RNA Tumor Viruses. In *Virus Infections*, pp. 223–54. L.C. Olson, ed. New York: Marcel Dekker.

Gleason, John A. 1986. Quarantine: An unreasonable solution to the AIDS dilemma. *Cincinnati Law Review* 55:217–35.

Goode, Stephen. 1987. After the loving comes the lawsuit. *Insight* March 9:66–67.

Gostin, Larry, and William J. Curran. 1987. Legal control measures for AIDS: Reporting requirements, surveillance, quarantine, and regulation of public meeting places. *American Journal of Public Health* 77:214–28.

Gross, Ludwig. 1970. *Oncogenic Viruses*. Oxford: Pergamon Press.

———. 1978. Viral Etiology of Cancer and Leukemia: A Look into the Past, Present and Future. *Cancer Research* 38:485–93.

———. 1980. The Search for Viruses as the Etiological Agents in Leukemia and Malignant Lymphomas: The Role of the Happy Accident and the Prepared Mind. *Cancer Research* 40:3405–7.

Guo, Hong-Guang; Franchini, Genoveffa; Collalti, Enrico, et al. 1987. Structure of the lone terminal repeat of simian lymphotropic virus type III (African green monkey) and its relatedness to that of HIV. *AIDS Research and Human Retroviruses* 3:177–83.

Hahn, Beatrice A.; Shaw, George M.; Taylor, Maria A.; et al. 1986. Genetic variation in HTLV-III/LAV over time in patients with AIDS or at risk for AIDS. *Science* 232:1548–53.

Hernandez, Ruben. 1986. Insuring herpes of mind. *New Times* 16:8.

Herpes in the workplace. 1984. *The Helper* 6:1–7.

Hitler, Adolf. 1939. *Mein Kampf*. London: Hurst and Blackett Ltd.

Ho, David D.; Pomerantz, Roger J.: and Joan C. Kaplan. 1987. Pathogenesis of infection with human immunodeficiency virus. *New England Journal of Medicine* 317:278–86.

Holland, John; Spindler, Katherine; Horodyski, Frank; et al. 1982. Rapid evolution of RNA genomes. *Science* 215:1577–85.

Kanki, P.J.; Barin, F.; M'Boup, S.; et al. 1986. New human t-lymphotropic retrovirus related to simian T-lymphotropic virus type III (STLV-III$_{AGM}$). *Science* 232:238–43.

Kant, Harold Sanford. 1985. The transmission of HTLV-III. *Journal of the American Medical Association* 254:1901.

Kreiss, Joan K.; Koech, Davy; Plummer, Francis A.; et al. 1986. AIDS virus infection in Nairobi prostitutes. *New England Journal of Medicine* 314:414–18.

Langone, John. 1985. Special Report: AIDS. *Discover* December: 28–53.

Leder, Aya; Swan, David; Ruddle, Frank; et al. 1981. Dispersion of ∝-like globin genes of the mouse to three different chromosomes. *Nature* 293:196–200.

Levy, J.A.; Hoffman, A.D.; Kramer, S.M.; et al. 1984. Isolation of Lymphocytopathic retroviruses from San Francisco patients with AIDS. *Science* 225:840–42.

Marx, Jean L. 1983. Acquired Immune Deficiency Syndrome Abroad. *Science* 222:998–99.

Masur, Henry; Michelis, Mary Ann; Wormser, Gary P.; et al. 1982. Opportunistic infection in previously healthy women: Initial manifestations of a community-acquired cellular immunodeficiency. *Annals of Internal Medicine* 97:533–39.

Matthews, Gene W., and Verla S. Neslund. 1987. The initial impact of AIDS on public health law in the United States. *Journal of the American Medical Association* 257:344–52.

McCombie, S. C. 1985. Measles eradication: The role of the anthropologist. *Atlatl* 5:23–40.

———. 1986. Cultural factors related to the epidemiology of viral hepatitis in a southwestern United States county. Ph.D. diss., University of Arizona, University Microfilms.

———. 1987. Folk flu and viral syndrome: An epidemiological perspective. *Social Science and Medicine* 25:987–93.

McNeill, William H. 1976. *Plagues and Peoples*. Garden City: Anchor Press.

Mims, Cedric. 1980. The Emergence of New Infectious Diseases. In *Changing Disease Patterns and Human Behavior*, pp. 231–50. N.F. Stanley and R.A. Joske, eds.

Nei, Masatoshi. 1987. *Molecular Evolutionary Genetics*. New York: Columbia University Press.

Newmark, Peter. 1987. Human and monkey virus puzzles. *Nature* 327:458.

Norman, Colin. 1985. Politics and science clash on African AIDS. *Science* 230:1140–42.

O'Brien, Carol. 1987. Arcadia physicians defend their position in AIDS/school dispute. *American Medical News* September 25:3–34.

Opportunistic diseases: A puzzling new syndrome afflicts homosexual men., 1981. *Time* December 21, 118:68.

Parran, Thomas. 1937. *Shadow on the Land: Syphilis*. New York: Reynal and Hitchcock.

Payne, A.M. 1955. Public health measures in the control of poliomyelitis. In *Poliomyelitis*. Geneva: World Health Organization.

Poiesz, B.J.; Ruscetti, F.W.; Gazdar, A.F.; et al. 1980. Isolation of Type C retrovirus particles from cultured and fresh lymphocytes of a patient with cutaneous T-cell leukemia. *Proceedings of the National Academy of Sciences* 77:7415–19.

Poiesz, B.J.; Ruscetti, F.W.; Reitz, M. S.; et al. 1981. Isolation of a new type C retrovirus (HTLV) in primary uncultured cells of a patient with Sezary T-cell leukemia. *Nature* 294:271–73.

Polk, B. Frank. 1985. Female-to-male transmission of AIDS. *Journal of the American Medical Association* 254:3177–78.

Popovic, M.; Sarin, P.S.; Gurroff, M.R.; et al. 1983. Isolation and Transmission of Human Retrovirus (Human T-cell leukemia virus). *Science* 219:856–59.

Popovic, M.; Sarngadharan, M.G.; Read, E.; and R.C. Gallo. 1984. Detection, isolation, and continuous production of cytopathic retroviruses (HTLV-III) from patients with AIDS and pre-AIDS. *Science* 224:497–500.

Pusey, Wm. Allen. 1915. *Syphilis as a modern problem*. Chicago: American Medical Association.

Rabson, A.B., and M.A. Martin. 1985. Molecular organization of the AIDS retrovirus. *Cell* 40:477–80.

Richards, Jon M.; Bedford, J. Michael; and Steven S. Witkin. 1984. Rectal insemination modifies immune responses in rabbits. *Science* 224:390–92.

Sande, Merle A. 1986. Transmission of AIDS: The case against casual contagion. *New England Journal of Medicine* 314:380–82.

Seale, John. 1985. Sexual transmission of AIDS virus. *British Journal of Hospital Medicine* August:71.

Sorlie, Paul D., and Ellen B. Gold. 1987. The effect of physician terminology preference on coronary heart disease mortality: An artifact uncovered by the 9th revision ICD. *American Journal of Public Health* 77:148–52.

U. S. Department of Health and Human Services. 1987. *Instructions for classifying the underlying cause of death, 1987*. Hyattsville: National Center for Health Statistics.

Van de Perre, Philippe; Rouvroy, Dominique; Lepage, Philippe; et al. 1984. Acquired immunodeficiency syndrome in Rwanda. *Lancet* July 14: 62–69.

Vianna, N.J. 1975. *Lymphoreticular Malignancies*. Baltimore: University Park Press.

Vogt, Markus W.; Witt, David J.; Craven, Donald E., et al. 1986. Isolation of HTLV-III/LAV from cervical secretions of women at risk for AIDS. *Lancet* March 8:525–27.

Weller, Thomas H. 1980. Contemporary Plagues and Social Progress. *Pediatrics* 66:458–61.

Winslow, Charles Edward-Amory. 1943. *The Conquest of Epidemic Disease*. New York: Hafner Publishing Company.

Wolf, John K. 1980. *Practical Clinical Neurology*. Garden City: Medical Examination Publishing Company.

# Chapter Three

## The Sick Role, Stigma, and Pollution: The Case of AIDS

### Michael D. Quam

## INTRODUCTION

The sudden emergence of a deadly infectious disease for which we have yet to develop any vaccine or cure, its rapid epidemic expansion on a global scale, and the fact that transmission of the infectious agent occurs during acts of sexual intimacy have created an extraordinary challenge to institutionalized concepts and behaviors regarding health. This chapter will focus on the phenomenon of AIDS in the culture and society of the United States, where the sociological and anthropological concepts to be discussed are clearly salient. Whether these concepts can be usefully applied to other sociocultural groups is an open question. In the course of our discussion we will move from one of the most established conceptual models in medical sociology, the Parsonian paradigm of the sick role, to the social psychological realm of the attribution of stigma, and finally to an aspect of cultural reality usually associated with non-Western societies, pollution and taboo. Our ultimate goal is a deeper understanding of the socio-cultural experience of the AIDS epidemic.

## THE SICK ROLE

In 1951, Talcott Parsons unveiled his monumental work of sociological theory, *The Social System*. Although he showed a good deal of interest in social psychology and psychodynamics, Parsons developed a model that was primarily functionalist with a heavy emphasis on the normative basis of social integration and stability. According to this view, the success of the social system in providing for the day-to-day needs of its members depends upon each person adequately performing their social roles, and each of us within the social system has normative role expectations of one another. Deviance from these expected role performances causes potential disruption of the social integration that is functionally necessary for the system's survival, and, therefore, any significant deviance inevitably and necessarily calls forth normative and socially structured ways to control and dispel such a disturbance. From Parsons's highly abstracted perspective, the social system experiences two generalized forms of deviance, distinguished by the deviant individual's degree of control over or responsibility for their behavior: the person who is capable of proper and constructive role performance but refuses to do so is criminal, while the person who is incapable of expected role performance is sick. In order to deal effectively with these deviations, the social system has developed two parallel ways of responding. Institutionally, criminal deviance is dealt with through the legal system, while sickness is treated within the medical system. Behaviorally, from a theoretical perspective both medicine and law use a similar approach to correction: segregate the deviant individual from the "normals," rehabilitate the individual, and then reintegrate them into the social system.[1]

One of the principal means of controlling deviance is to develop relevant role expectations even for those who fail to perform "normal" roles. These special deviant roles carry within their script the expectation that the individual will behave in a minimally disruptive manner and according to rules that are at least functionally congruent with the dominant norms and values. The sick role, with its attendant rights and responsibilities, is socially structured to control the spread of dysfunctional behavior (for example, if others see that being labelled "sick" enables one to avoid work, they may begin malingering), and to end (or cure) dysfunctional behavior in the individual. The script for the sick role is composed of four major aspects, two rights and two responsibilities. First, the individual is exempted from normal role obligations, that is, is not expected to meet the routine expectations and needs of others. Second, by social definition within this role the person is not held responsible for his or her condition. To balance these two special rights, a third component of the role is the expectation that the sick person will view his or her state of illness as undesirable, and fourth, will seek out and cooperate with those who are technically competent and socially assigned to the task of healing, that is, medical professionals. In other words, the sick person is expected to do everything one can to get well as soon as possible (Parsons 1951:436–37).

Since its initial formulation, the sick role has been a central concept in the sociology of medicine (see major reviews by Twaddle 1979 and Levine and Kozloff 1978). It is discussed in virtually every medical sociology textbook and examined analytically for its usefulness and validity. Empirical studies have yielded conflicting results on whether the concept as delineated by Parsons (1951,1958, 1975) accurately reflects the normative role expectations regarding sickness actually held by people in American society. But most commentators agree that as an ideal type, which was Parsons's original intent, the sick role concept has been helpful in examining sickness behavior and the social response to sickness.

For our purposes, we will focus on three critical problems in applying the sick role to the phenomenon of AIDS. We begin by asking a question commonly posed in the empirical application of this concept: Under what circumstances does a person enter the sick role? As Mechanic (1978:273–87) has pointed out, illness may be self-defined or other-defined, and although in an individual case these two points of view may be compatible, considerable differences of perception and behavioral response can arise. Several of the variables that influence the response to illness have to do with symptoms, that is, the "visibility or recognizability of symptoms," the perceived severity and seriousness of the physical or behavioral deviation, the "frequency and persistence" of symptoms, and the ability of the individual or others to tolerate the discomfort and disruption of normal routines. In addition, the availability of treatment and the basic medical awareness of those affected can also determine whether a condition is treated as an illness and whether the affected individual enters the sick role.

AIDS is certainly considered a serious illness, but when is a person considered to "have AIDS?" No doubt, someone who is medically diagnosed as meeting the Centers for Disease Control definition of full-blown AIDS will be universally recognized as meeting the social definition of sickness and accorded the release from normal role expectations. But the person with AIDS may not wish to be placed in the sick role. If the person is not at the moment feeling ill, is not hospitalized, and is capable of carrying on most normal routines and roles, the sick role may be inappropriate. This anomalous situation can provoke great anxiety in the person with AIDS and especially in others who are confused about how they should respond to the person. Contradictions in self-defined and other-defined illness become even more pronounced regarding the person who is HIV-infected but has no visible symptoms and has experienced no illness. The infected asymptomatic person may feel perfectly capable of performing normal role expectations, but some such activities would be medically precluded because they create the risk of transmission of infection to others, that is, unsafe sexual activities and exposure to blood. Such a proscription can be very disruptive, even in the absence of any actual symptoms, to intimate relationships. Beyond the circle of intimacy, the popular perception is that the infected person, no matter what symptoms are or are not evident, "has AIDS." The social interactional meaning of this ascription is that the future of the infected person is death from this terrible disease, and that the person is dangerous to others. Most people assume that the infected person should be under a doctor's care (indeed, the clinics that test for infection recommend to those who test positive that they consult a physician), even though the disease is also perceived to be incurable. And certainly there is a widespread and recurrent demand that infected persons be relieved of obligations, or perhaps deprived of opportunities, for normal[2] social interactions and role performance. Many people insist that asymptomatic HIV-infected persons be considered sick, because they are incapable of performing "normal" role expectations through "normal" social interaction without putting others in what is perceived as danger. To this end, many people continue to insist that the identity of those who are infected should be discovered and revealed.

Our second problem with the sick role model has to do with the obligation to seek technically competent help and cooperate in treatment, that is, to try to get well. The criticism that this aspect of the sick role cannot be applied to chronic and especially incurable disease has been made many times since it was so effectively stated by Gallagher (1976). Without a cure and with only minimally effective treatment, AIDS is a prime example of this problem. Many AIDS patients are cooperating fully with their doctors' orders and even making extra efforts to heal themselves through "wellness" activities such as dietary regimens and stress reduction. Many have eagerly sought to enroll in experimental drug trials conducted by technically competent medical scientists. Because AIDS is still incurable by these technically competent healers, many persons with AIDS have also sought out alternative remedies, be it experimenting with drugs that are not officially approved or looking for supernatural help through religious practices. Even if treatment modalities become more effective in prolonging life, persons with AIDS will not be fully rehabilitated to socially functional "normality" as envisioned in the Parsonian model, nor will they be reintegrated into "normal" social interaction and role performance, for, as noted earlier, the "normals" consider persons with AIDS to be incurably dangerous. Thus, because their dysfunction is incurable, persons with AIDS become permanent players of the sick role, not the kind of situation that Parsons described. However, in keeping with a broad functionalist analysis, this situation of ever-increasing numbers of people, many of them in their early adult years, becoming very seriously ill and requiring extensive and expensive care is creating an alarming burden of social dysfunction.

In attempting to apply the sick role model to AIDS, the most complex issues arise regarding the sick person's responsibility for his or her condition. Twaddle (1979:44–45) notes that Parsons intended this part of the model to refer to the continuation of the illness, not its onset. In other words, once the person is sick, no matter what the etiology of the illness, the individual is not held responsible for curing him or herself, that is, the sick person is "helpless." But as Twaddle (1979:57–58) also admits, this particular aspect of the model is ambiguous even in Parsons's own formulation (Parsons 1951:440).

Parsons has based his model on the concept of sickness being deviant, and in some significant respects analogous to crime. Friedson (1970:205–23) focuses on this portion of the model and uses an alternative concept of deviance to indicate the shortcomings in Parson's theory. Discarding a functionalist approach, Friedson develops a situational theory of illness as deviance:

What is called deviance in human society is something that breaks a social rule or norm. It may exist as an act or attribute independently of social rules or norms—as breaking a window exists independently of laws and breaking a leg exists independently of medicine—but it cannot exist *as social deviance* independently of the social rules or norms that assign the *meaning* of deviance to the act or attribute. In this sense, deviance is created by social rules and cannot exist independently of social life. . . . It follows that the *perception and designation* of deviance is at least as important as the actual *act or behavior* in determining whether the social role of deviance will be assumed or not. . . . The etiology of deviance as a social role does not thus lie in the individual "deviant" so much as in the social process of creating rules that make acts or attributes deviant, of labeling people as deviant or offenders, and of managing those labeled as deviants. (Freidson 1970:217)

Illness is a particular kind of social deviance, "stemming from current . . . conceptions of what disease is, limited perhaps by whatever few biological facts are universally recognized, and ordered by organizations and occupations devoted to defining, uncovering, and managing illness" (ibid.:223), but it is not neatly divorced from the general moral considerations with which all forms of deviance are imbued. And it is with this consideration in mind that Freidson takes on the issue of responsibility.

Friedson has shifted the focus of analysis from the ill person as deviant to the societal response which determines who is deviant and in what ways rules have been broken. A critical qualitative variable in this response is whether blame is ascribed to the individual. When an illness is perceived as sufficiently serious and the ill person is held blameless for their deviation, then legitimacy is also ascribed and the sick role is entered unconditionally. But if the illness is perceived to be the result of some serious deviation from social rules and norms, then the ill person may be denied the sick role and instead treated as a criminal. For example, sexually transmitted diseases are medically labeled as illness, but since they are the result of non-monogamous sexual relations[3], which according to idealized American moral standards are acts of moral deviance, they are illegitimate and cannot be used as the reason for entering the sick role. In fact, historically Americans have treated those who are infected or even suspected of being infected as criminals, employing punitive measures such as mass quarantines and messages of moral condemnation to try to control this particular disease threat (Brandt 1985).

AIDS as a disease which is sexually transmitted is clearly included in this category of illnesses that are considered illegitimate.[4] Indeed, debates about disease control often take on a rhetorical tone more appropriate to crime control. Demands for "tough" measures of disease control are voiced repeatedly by public officials, common citizens, and even some members of the medical profession. Civil liberties concerns regarding AIDS are often viewed in the same light as "coddling criminals."

An internal Justice Department memorandum urges officials to "polarize the debate" on such key legal issues as drugs, AIDS, obscenity and the death penalty and to seek confrontation instead of consensus in the remaining days of the Reagan administration. . . . The memorandum says, "AIDS is not a civil rights or privacy issue, but one of public health and safety." It recommends that the department press lawsuits that seek to counter "the privacy advocates who challenge AIDS testing." (Administration Memo 1988)

Disease control programs requiring mandatory testing and isolation, with much of the implementation done through the law enforcement system, are repeatedly proposed. The popular imagination is fueled by media accounts of a new kind of dangerous celebrity figure. In a public television special report, a poverty-stricken and disoriented young black man with AIDS says that he has been shuttling around the country by bus and earning a meager living through male prostitution. In a best-selling book on the AIDS crisis (Shilts 1987), a Canadian airline steward with AIDS, apparently devastatingly handsome and possessing an enormous appetite for gay sexual partners, becomes posthumously notorious as the man who may have spread the infection coast-to-coast while denying his own illness. These stories feed the belief that infected people will behave without any regard for the safety of others, and even deliberately infect others. In the 1987 legislative session, one of the Illinois legislators claimed that some infected persons were engaging in "blood terrorism" by donating at blood centers. Most recently, the U.S. military has tried and convicted two infected individuals because they had unprotected sex with partners who were not informed of the danger involved. (AIDS-infected Soldier 1987). Clearly, in the case of AIDS, the culturally defined line between sickness and crime is blurred. The illegitimacy of the actions that lead to infection is a moral stain that stays with the person even when one would otherwise be eligible for entry into the sick role. Their personal responsibility for the illness, and the perceived lack of responsibility toward others, make the situation culturally ambiguous, and the social response is therefore ambivalent.

## STIGMA

In his critique of Parsons, Friedson (1970:235–40) explores the phenomenon of stigma as a dynamic element in the way we respond to certain illnesses.

For "normal" illness, many normal obligations are suspended; only the obligation to seek help is incurred. But in the case of the stigmatized, a complex variety of new obligations is incurred. Whereas in the former instance the burden of adjustment (through permissiveness and support) lies on the "normals" around the sick person, the burden in the latter lies on the stigmatized person when he is around "normals." (ibid.:236)

According to Goffman (1963:11), in the original Greek meaning of the term, *stigma* referred to "bodily signs designed to expose something unusual and bad about the moral status of the signifier," although today stigma "is applied more to the disgrace itself than to the bodily evidence of it." In either case—and both are applicable to AIDS—the individual is marked by a trait that is "discredited" or, if hidden, is "discreditable" (ibid.:14). When personal responsibility for the stigma can be imputed to the individual, the severity of stigmatization increases (Jones 1984:58–60).

Several studies (cited in Jones 1984) have established fear as a highly salient feature of stigma. In an example directly relevant to the case of AIDS, Bobys and Laner (1979) found "ex-homosexuals"[5] were stigmatized primarily because they were perceived as "dangerous." Goffman (1963:15) is even more direct when he says, "By definition, of course, we believe the person with a stigma is not quite human." The possibility of contagion seems to be the basis for some of this fear. Goffman (ibid.:43, 64, 147) alludes to the tendency of stigma to spread from the stigmatized to close associates, ironically labelling this phenomenon "courtesy stigma." Of course, people with communicable diseases are at least temporarily avoided because of the real danger of contagion, but this social reaction may also extend to care-givers and close associates. When it takes on the form of stigma, the avoidance becomes shunning and is much more widespread. Remarkably, the stigma of danger from communicable diseases extends even to noncommunicable diseases and disabilities (Jones 1984:69–71). And the phenomenon of "courtesy stigma" is based on ideas of at least symbolic contagion.

The ascription of stigma to any condition arises out of the symbol system within a culture, and, like other symbolic acts, follows a logic within which relationships are more emotional than rational. Not too long ago in a hospital in rural Illinois, an elderly woman patient adamantly refused a medically necessary blood transfusion because, she said, she feared she might become a "homosexual." Her confusion regarding cause and effect is better understood as illuminating some of her culture's deepest fears regarding the disease and stigmatization of AIDS. Because of its associations with nonmonogamous, and especially homosexual, sex and with intravenous drug use, activities that are considered immoral by some and in some venues even illegal, any contact with the symbolic or real bearers of this disease must be avoided. Persons who are known to be infected have been shunned by their closest friends and family members, have been evicted from their dwellings, and have been dismissed from their employment. The extreme stigmatization of AIDS derives in part from its associations with deviant behaviors but has also, as a sort of added "courtesy stigma," increased the rejection of those who are thought to be "at risk" of being infected. The "danger" they pose has given rise to an increase in acts of interpersonal violence against gay men and lesbians (Meislin 1986). In response, health professionals trying to stem the tide of disease through the usual practices of disease control and health care have found it necessary to impose airtight measures of confidentiality in their contacts with infected persons.

Fear and stigma have also charged the political atmosphere surrounding governmental efforts to address this epidemic (Shilts 1987). During the first five years of the epidemic while thousands of cases were appearing, the president of the United States did not publicly mention the name of this dreaded disease. The federal health bureaucracy was forced to make internal reallocations for AIDS programs because it was politically impossible to secure adequate funding for the research and prevention programs they knew were needed. Seven years into the epidemic, the chairperson of the Presidential Commission on the HIV Epidemic admitted that "there has not been a national strategy" to combat the disease (Boffey 1988).

The barrier to action seems to be the inevitable association with stigmatized behavior that health education and risk reduction activities entails. Those who would limit such efforts to simple messages of moral condemnation and exhortation have the cultural imprimatur of stigma avoidance as their foundation. Teaching people in plain and common terms how to avoid infection, for example, use condoms and disinfect needles, seems implicitly to condone the stigmatized "life-styles" that involve high risk behavior. And because the stigma itself is contagious, the logic of symbolic associations dictates that the behaviors themselves must also be contagious. Americans have used the term "epidemic" to characterize the growth of the drug use problem, and even before AIDS, gays were thought to be dangerous and were often forbidden to be school teachers, as it was feared a gay teacher would corrupt the youngsters in his charge. Gays are still excluded from the ranks of the military.

But how and why would such corruption occur? Apparently, in most people's minds these forbidden activities, namely homosexuality and drug use, must be pleasurable (albeit, "perversely" so), and therefore one could be seduced into them. The symbolic connection between sex and drugs is borne out in the testimony of intravenous drug users themselves. They describe their first experience as similar to their initiation into sex, and needle-sharing partners are also frequently sexual partners (Des Jarlais, Friedman, and Strug 1986). Furthermore, in the popular image, one shot of heroin is enough to make one an addict. As with drugs, so with sex. Even if actual addiction is not the result, and even if the person abandons those deviant activities, the stigma of the behavior becomes a permanent part of the person's identity (Freidson 1970:236), staining one's character forever.

Among some Christian sects, AIDS is seen as another example of the biblical admonition that "the wages of sin is death." For many Americans such an idea has meaning derived from messages they internalized during their childhood. Their parents and other parental authorities warned them that if they succumbed to the "appetites of the flesh," they would suffer dire consequences. Now AIDS has appeared to fulfill such prophecies. And even if liberal tolerance dictates acceptance of "alternative life-styles," the fearsome fact of death remains. Many people have seen or read descriptions of persons with AIDS. The body is wasting away, the person disintegrating, losing mental abilities, losing physical powers, losing any reason or ability to go on. That this terrible death has befallen a person in the prime of life (most persons with AIDS are under 50) makes it even more threatening. Death at an early age is itself stigmatized, for the dying person reminds the witnesses of their own vulnerability (Jones 1984:66–67).

The AIDS stigma of deviance and death has influenced the delivery of health care services to persons who are infected (Quam 1986). At the local level many physicians refuse to have their names placed on a referral list for patients with HIV-related disease. The issue was brought into the national limelight when a prominent surgeon in Milwaukee refused to operate on an HIV-infected patient and counseled other physicians to exercise the same judgment (Heart Surgeon 1987). The debate over this kind of discriminatory behavior has continued inside the American Medical Association (Pear 1987). The dentistry profession is even more intransigent. Despite the professional rhetoric of commitment to service, in many communities it is nearly impossible to find a dentist who will serve a patient known to be infected (Quam 1986). Dentists argue that they will lose their technical staff and their other patients if it is suspected that they are working with infected persons. Some dentists and physicians who avoid contact with infected persons claim the dangers involved are not acceptable to their family members.

Nurses have reported the subtle distinctions drawn in hospital care between AIDS patients who are "innocent victims," infants who were infected by their mothers and adults who were infected through transfusions, and those who are by implication guilty, those who became infected through sexual or drug use activities. The amount of "sentimental work" done (Strauss et al. 1985)[6], the quickness of response to patient requests for assistance, the interaction with the patient's family and friends can all be affected by this moral evaluation.

It should be noted, however, that the fear element in AIDS stigma can override any moral discrimination, as evidenced by the rejection of school children who are infected through the use of blood products to control another disease, hemophilia. Some parents and school officials have proposed testing all children with hemophilia for HIV infection or simply banning them from school. In a nationally publicized case in Florida, the family of two such children was forced to leave town after threats of violence and an arson fire in their home (Family in AIDS Case 1987). This attack was a shocking indication of the emotional depths touched by the fear of AIDS. To understand these extreme reactions, we need to add some depth to our conceptual framework.

## POLLUTION

As one who has suffered the disease and stigma of cancer, Susan Sontag writes with great passion and insight about the way Americans symbolically construct and respond to disease. "Any disease that is treated as a mystery and acutely enough feared will be felt to be morally, if not literally, contagious. . . . Contact with someone afflicted with a disease regarded as a mysterious malevolency inevitably feels like a trespass; worse, like a violation of a taboo" (Sontag 1978:5–6). AIDS is universally characterized as both mysterious and malevolent. One of the most common phrases one hears regarding AIDS, even from medical scientists, is "we know so little about it." And infection with the virus that causes AIDS is felt to be a defilement, a violation of the person, even an assault (in several legal jurisdictions people have been charged with assault because it was believed they exposed someone to infection [Deadly Weapon 1987; Boorstin 1987; Johnson 1987]).

These intense feelings bring to mind the kind of fear associated with beliefs regarding pollution. As Mary Douglas (1966), our leading contemporary theorist on this subject, has pointed out, pollution is fundamentally the result of contact with "dirt." Contemporary European and North American ideas of defilement by dirt seem to focus on aesthetics and hygiene: "Our idea of dirt is dominated by the knowledge of pathogenic organisms" (Douglas 1966:35). In the case of AIDS, the orifices of the body where the virus enters, at least when it is sexually transmitted, are symbolically considered "dirty": the anus because of feces, the vagina where menstrual blood flows, and the penis because of urination, ejaculation, and penetration of the "dirty" vagina or anus. But feelings regarding this kind of dirt run even deeper. The multivocal and dialectical nature of symbolic realities is evident in American thinking about AIDS. The fact that two primary vital elements, semen and blood, should be the carriers of pollution and death increases the sense of the polluting power of AIDS and the fear of the disease.

At a more basic level, dirt is "matter out of place, . . . the by-product of a systematic ordering and classification of matter, in so far as ordering involves rejecting inappropriate elements" (Douglas 1966:39). Something that does not fit in the classification system is anomalous, and one of the ways of dealing with anomalous events or elements is to label them dangerous. So dirt is disorder that is dangerous. As Douglas (1966:113) puts it, "A polluting person is always in the wrong. He has developed some wrong condition or simply crossed some line which should not have been crossed and this displacement unleashes danger for someone." Furthermore, danger beliefs are used in order to enforce the moral code:

The laws of nature are dragged in to sanction the moral code: this kind of disease is caused by adultery, that by incest . . . certain moral beliefs are upheld and certain social rules defined by beliefs in dangerous contagion, as when the glance or touch of an adulterer is held to bring illness to his neighbors or his children. (Douglas 1966:3)

Within American culture and society, gays and intravenous drug users are anomalous, they do not fit "normal" social categories. Such persons have crossed some line, some boundary of "nature" that makes them less than human and essentially dangerous. Now, with the advent of AIDS, gays and intravenous drug users are epidemiologically labeled the "high risk groups." Through a linguistic double entendre, unintended by the epidemiologists, the culturally defined danger these groups pose for the "normals" seems to be medically confirmed.

Speaking more concretely, how is this pollution danger experienced? Let us once again draw an analogy with cancer. Sontag (1978:5, 8, 13) says cancer is "an illness experienced as a ruthless, secret invasion." The cancer patient is invaded by "alien cells," and the disease "works slowly and insidiously." Furthermore, cancer is "obscene," that is, "ill-omened, abominable, repugnant to the senses." An obvious biomedical connection exists between cancer and AIDS. One of the most common opportunistic diseases associated with AIDS is Kaposi's sarcoma, a tissue cancer that is manifest in spots and lesions, literally marking its sufferers and thus being repugnant and stigmatizing. And, of course, AIDS also works slowly and insidiously.

Parsons (1951), in his analysis of the American medical system, discusses the inviolability of the body as an important emotionally loaded value in American culture, noting how people are squeamish about needles even when used for medically necessary injections. By symbolic analogy, the virus that causes AIDS infects a person by penetrating the body somehow, and that biological fact is felt as an invasion and violation of the body. Epidemiologically, the principal identified modes of HIV transmission are, in fact, acts of penetration; culturally, they are acts of violation. Penile penetration of the rectum is considered "abnormal" within the dominant culture, even "unnatural" (albeit that it is not uncommon in heterosexual intercourse), and thus it is violating. This notion is reinforced by popular tales of violent homosexual rape in prisons and by medical explanations of why rectal intercourse is especially risky for viral transmission, the rectum is not built for this kind of use and the walls are traumatized/ruptured/torn by this unusual friction. Injecting illegal drugs that alter the person's thinking and feeling is also seen as a violation of the person. Even though this violation is self-generated, the loss of self-control through addiction is frightening and is often characterized as suicidal. For those who do not knowingly put themselves at risk through these particular acts, the fear that they might still somehow become infected by polluting contact is a fear of violating bodily penetration: symbolically, a fear of rape.

Both concretely and metaphorically, the body is often the locus of pollution. Douglas (1966:115–21) states this point very clearly.

The body is a model which can stand for any bounded system. Its boundaries can represent any boundaries which are threatened or precarious. . . . [We can] see in the body a symbol of society, and . . . see the powers and dangers credited to social structure reproduced in small on the human body. . . . Why should body margins be thought to be specially invested with power and danger? . . . [A]ll margins are dangerous. If they are pulled this way or that the shape of fundamental experience is altered. Any structure of ideas is vulnerable at its margins. We should expect the orifices of the body to symbolize its specially vulnerable points. Matter issuing from them is marginal stuff of the most obvious kind. Spittle, blood, milk, urine, faeces or tears by simply issuing forth have traversed the boundary of the body.

To understand what precarious social or cultural margins are being mirrored in pollution beliefs regarding the body, Douglas advises, we must "try to argue back from the known dangers of society to the known selection of bodily themes and try to recognize what appositeness is there" (1966:121). As an exercise in such analysis, let us consider the body pollution of AIDS.

What vulnerable social boundaries are being symbolically evoked by the threat of AIDS? The first that immediately comes to mind is personal safety. With rising rates of street crime and home invasion—armed robbery, assault, rape, and murder—Americans have come to fear the dangerous stranger. This pervasive sense of physical insecurity is the result of the failure of social community to provide some kind of embracing protection, and the failure of the police powers to protect the vulnerable individual from increasing risk of violent attack. With a growing awareness of domestic violence comes the fear of the dangerous intimate. People sense a failure in the institutions of courtship, marriage, and the family to protect the individual from harm by someone with whom they have been intimate, that is, let down their self-protective guard and become vulnerable.

The social apparatus of science and technology in which Americans have invested so much faith is also now suspect. The failure of the technological experts to protect people from the experiment, procedure, or complex machine that goes wrong and unleashes an uncontrollable life-threatening danger is the theme of many popular novels, movies, and television dramas. A recent paperback thriller, *June Mail* (Warmbold 1986), is based on the premise that AIDS is the result of a U.S. biological warfare experiment, a conspiracy theory that has enjoyed wide circulation in the Third World and in some U.S. circles. Attempts by public health officials to argue against such speculation are undermined by an erosion of confidence in the competence and integrity of the people who control advanced technology. Recent disasters in nuclear power (Three Mile Island and Chernobyl), the space program (the explosion of *Challenger*), and toxic chemical production (Union Carbide in Bhopal and in West Virginia) belie the experts' soothing assurances of safety.

A second set of social and cultural margins is also precarious. Ambiguities and contradictions have developed in the moral code, especially reflected in the conflict between the Protestant ethic of self-denial and the impulsiveness of hedonism. Americans envy those who have led a hedonistic life, not followed the rules of good citizenship and instead crossed some boundaries for the sake of self-gratification (witness the national fascination with the indiscretions of celebrities). But they find their own repressed desires very frightening, because if they were to act on such impulses, the resulting disruption would threaten their social security and personal identity. For most Americans, to work hard and be law-abiding is to be a good person in the eyes of others and in one's own eyes, but it is also to be a drone, to deny oneself the life of glamour, adventure, and danger that is held up for admiration and envy in images that bombard the public daily from television, movies, magazines, even from the evening news. In talking with Americans about AIDS, one is frequently struck by a tone of satisfaction underlying the expressions of fear. They seem to be saying that finally something undeniably awful has occurred that makes clear the dangers of self-indulgence.

AIDS is a nearly perfect metaphor for all of these insecurities and ambivalences. Both social and personal control seem to be breaking down. In Yeats's (1956:184–85) famous lines,

> Turning and turning in the widening gyre
> The falcon cannot hear the falconer;
> Things fall apart; the centre cannot hold;
> Mere anarchy is loosed upon the world,
> The blood-dimmed tide is loosed, and everywhere
> The ceremony of innocence is drowned;
> The best lack all conviction, while the worst
> Are full of passionate intensity.

And through it all the person has been left defenseless. Now Americans are plagued by a disease that attacks the very defense system of the body, is borne by bodily fluids, is inflicted through the violation of the body, and destroys the person. Small wonder that such a threat gives rise to feelings of pollution and to demands for pollution control.

## CONCLUSION

The realization that AIDS is evoking feelings of pollution within American culture only deepens the dilemma of how to deal with this very serious epidemic. In many non-Western cultures where pollution beliefs have great salience for the organization of social life, the problem of defilement can be solved through rituals of cleansing. But in the West where the phenomenon of personal and interpersonal pollution is greatly attenuated, we have abandoned such rituals[7] and are left with our physicians as the only ones who can rid us of the consequences of unclean acts. These high priests of biomedicine are helpless in the face of AIDS.

The extreme fear and the punitive response to AIDS are reminiscent of the emotional and social upheaval created by the advent of racial integration in schools, restaurants, housing, workplaces, etc. Then, as now with AIDS, contact with stigmatized minority persons was felt by the majority to be a violation of a pollution boundary, and the fear was frequently acted out in violence against the minority. The analogy can be further drawn: the marks of stigma were in the body (racism is a spurious biological ideology) and fear-inducing stereotypes of unbridled sexuality, disease, and other physical dangers abounded. This analogy is filled with disturbing portent as the AIDS epidemic is increasingly associated with minority persons.

Finally, the imputing of personal responsibility for their condition to persons with AIDS may be just an especially dramatic example of a trend that began many decades ago in American medical culture. The publication of the Flexner Report in 1910 is generally viewed as a watershed event in the organization and ideology of American medicine. The establishment of scientific medicine with its focus on the individual both in treatment and in research "had the effect of making the individual responsible for his or her own health, and, in effect, of taking this responsibility away from society" (Berliner 1975:577). Contemporary concerns over the costs of health care have given rise to a modern version of prevention, one which emphasizes the deleterious effects of individual "life-styles." John Knowles, the late president of the Rockefeller Foundation, made the point quite directly:

[C]ontrol of the present major health problems in the United States depends directly on modification of the individual's behavior and habit of living. . . . I believe the idea of a 'right' to health should be replaced by the idea of an individual moral obligation to preserve one's own health—a public duty if you will. The individual then has the "right" to expect help with information, accessible services of good quality, and minimal financial barriers. (1977:59,61)

This perspective is an ideological foundation for denying individuals who engage in risky behavior access to "good quality" health care services and even to health information. The advocates of individual responsibility seem uninterested in the complexities of individual motivation or the role of cultural conditioning in the shaping of behavior. They seem to assume a uniformly high degree of autonomous individual control over one's life circumstances, denying the relevance of gender, social class, or racial caste in determining the parameters of individual choice. The very term "life-style" has the connotation of free consumer choice, perhaps in keeping with an implicit emphasis on health as a marketplace commodity. If this ideological trend continues to gain credence in American culture, the sick role will become increasingly irrelevant and may be replaced with a very different configuration, something we might call the "at-risk" role. This change in the way Americans perceive and respond to illness will not be confined to persons with AIDS.

## NOTES

1. In terms of our interests, it is worth noting that the necessity to isolate the deviant implies the danger of contagion.

2. Throughout this chapter the term "normal" is used in the social psychological sense of that which is culturally prescribed and expected. Thus, "normal" connotes both the dominant values of the society and the most frequent behavior. In no case is "normal" meant to connote "natural" or "universally good."

3. Although in the strictest sense "monogamy" is a form of single-partner marriage,

in this context "nonmonogamous" refers to sexual relations, whether or not marriage is involved, with more than one person.

4. From a biomedical and epidemiologic perspective, the status of AIDS as a sexually transmitted disease is ambiguous. Although sexual transmission accounts for the majority of reported cases, other nonsexual modes of parenteral transmission are also significant. Thus, many public health officials have been reluctant to categorize HIV infection as a sexually transmitted disease. Nevertheless, in the popular perception and in much AIDS education this identification is obvious.

5. The term "ex-homosexual" may strike some readers as rather odd. Bobys and Laner (1979) are referring to men who formerly were exclusively or primarily homosexual in their sexual behavior but who have subsequently become exclusively heterosexual in their sexual behavior.

6. Strauss et al. (1985), describe "sentimental work" within health care as interaction with the patient as a person, including knowledge and sensitivity to the patient's relationships with family members and other loved ones, awareness of fears and anxieties, and so forth.

7. Some observers of American culture have noted an emphasis on cleanliness, especially evident in frequent hand-washing, bathing, and use of various soaps, detergents, and disinfectants. Certainly, the American belief in the germ theory is obvious in behavior. But none of this behavior has the peculiar qualities of ritual as delineated by Turner (1969) or Rappaport (1979).

## REFERENCES

Administration Memo Urges Confrontation on Legal Issues. 1988. *New York Times*, Feb. 27:Y15.

AIDS-infected Soldier Is Sentenced. 1987. *New York Times*, Dec. 4:Y17.

Army Sergeant Pleads Guilty of Infecting a G.I. with AIDS. 1987. *New York Times*, Dec. 17:Y15.

Berliner, H. S. 1975. A Larger Perspective on the Flexner Report. *International Journal of Health Services* 5:573–92.

Bobys, R. S., and M. R. Laner. 1979. On the Stability of Stigmatization: The Case of Ex-homosexual Males. *Archives of Sexual Behavior* 8:247–61.

Boffey, P. M. 1988. Panel on AIDS Urges Growth in Health Care. *New York Times*, Feb. 25:Y1.

Boorstin, R. O. 1987. AIDS Spread Brings Action in the Courts. *New York Times*, June 19:Y1.

Brandt, A. 1985. *No Magic Bullet: A Social History of Venereal Disease in the United States.* New York: Oxford University Press.

Deadly Weapon in AIDS Verdict Is Inmate's Teeth. 1987. *New York Times*, June 25:Y11.

Des Jarlais, D. C.; S. R. Friedman; and D. Strug. 1986. AIDS and Needle-sharing within the IV-drug Use Subculture. In *Social Dimensions of AIDS: Method and Theory*, pp. 111–25. D. A. Feldman and T. M. Johnson, eds. New York: Praeger.

Douglas, M. 1966. *Purity and Danger: An Analysis of the Concepts of Pollution and Taboo.* London: Routledge and Kegan Paul.

Family in AIDS Case Quits Florida Town after House Burns. 1987. *New York Times*, August 30:Y1.

Freidson, E. 1970. *Profession of Medicine: A Study of the Sociology of Applied Knowledge.* New York: Harper and Row.

Gallagher, E. B. 1976. Lines of Reconstruction and Extension in the Parsonian Sociology of Illness. *Social Science and Medicine* 10:207–18.

Goffman, E. 1963. *Stigma: Notes on the Management of Spoiled Identity.* Harmondsworth, England: Penquin.

Heart Surgeon Won't Operate on Victims of AIDS. 1987. *New York Times,* March 13:Y11.

Johnson, K. 1987. New York Police Say Suspect Bit Officer and Claimed to Have AIDS. *New York Times,* June 10:Y16.

Jones, E. E., et al. 1984. *Social Stigma: The Psychology of Marked Relationships.* New York: W. H. Freeman.

Knowles, J. H. 1977. The Responsibility of the Individual. *Daedalus* 106(1):57:80.

Levine, S., and M. A. Kozloff. 1978. The Sick Role: Assessment and Overview. *Annual Review of Sociology* 4:317–43.

Mechanic, D. 1978. *Medical Sociology.* 2d ed. New York: The Free Press.

Meislin, R. J. 1986. AIDS Fears Said to Increase Prejudice Against Homosexuals. *New York Times,* Jan. 21:Y10.

Parsons, T. 1951. *The Social System.* New York: The Free Press.

———. 1958. Definitions of Health and Illness in the Light of American Values and Social Structure. In *Patients, Physicians and Illness.* E. G. Jaco, ed. Glencoe, Ill.: The Free Press.

———. 1975. The Sick Role and the Role of the Physician Reconsidered. *Milbank Memorial Fund Quarterly* 53:257–78.

Pear, R. 1987. A.M.A. Rules that Doctors Are Obligated to Treat AIDS. *New York Times,* Nov. 13:Y10.

Quam, M.D. 1986. Community Preparation for AIDS. Paper presented at the American Anthropological Association Annual Meeting, Philadelphia, Pa.

Rappaport, R. A. 1979. The Obvious Aspects of Ritual. In *Ecology, Meaning, and Religion,* pp. 173–221. Berkeley, CA: North Atlantic Books.

Shilts, R. 1987. *And the Band Played On: Politics, People, and the AIDS Epidemic.* New York: St. Martin's.

Sontag, S. 1978. *Illness as Metaphor.* New York: Vintage.

Strauss, A., et al. 1985. *Social Organization of Medical Work.* Chicago: University of Chicago Press.

Turner, V. 1969. *The Ritual Process.* Chicago: Aldine.

Twaddle, A. C. 1979. *Sickness Behavior and the Sick Role.* Cambridge, Mass.: Schenkman.

Warmbold, J. 1986. *June Mail.* Sag Harbor, N.Y.: The Permanent Press.

Yeats, W. B. 1956. *The Collected Poems of W. B. Yeats.* New York: Macmillan.

# Chapter Four

## Assessing Viral, Parasitic, and Sociocultural Cofactors Affecting HIV–1 Transmission in Rwanda

### Douglas A. Feldman

Penile-vaginal intercourse, based upon various research studies, is clearly the major mode of human immunodeficiency virus, type one (HIV–1) transmission in Rwanda (Carael et al. 1985; Clumeck et al. 1984; Feldman 1986a, 1989; Feldman et al. 1987; Feldman and Taylor, forthcoming; Lepage et al. 1985; Van de Perre et al. 1984). Other modes of transmission undoubtedly contribute to the spread of HIV in that central African country. Some HIV infected persons have been exposed through a blood transfusion, some undoubtedly through male homosexual activity, some probably through heterosexual anal intercourse, some perhaps through unsterilized needles used during medical injections, and some possibly through infected razor blades used during therapeutic scarification. But these are certainly relatively minor modes of HIV transmission compared with penile-vaginal intercourse (Lepage et al. 1986; Van de Perre, Kanyamupira et al. 1985). Ethnographic and additional epidemiologic research is urgently needed to assess precisely what roles these minor modes of transmission play in augmenting the overall pattern of HIV seroconversion in Rwanda and other African nations.

Based upon conversations with several traditional healers in Rwanda during research conducted by the author in 1985, what Western medicine calls "AIDS" is relatively new to Rwanda. It probably entered into that country from elsewhere in central Africa during the middle or late 1970s. The lack of stored sera from before that time period has precluded the possibility of an investigation into the question of whether HIV existed in a presumably nonpathogenic state before the mid-1970s in Rwanda. An examination of stored sera from 1959 in Kinshasa, Zaire has found one sample out of 818 to be HIV–1 positive by both repeated ELISA and Western blot (Nahmias et al. 1986). However, it is uncertain whether that one sample was a biological false positive test result or not, or—indeed—whether it was reflective of illness in the infected person.

Although it is not known when HIV first entered the United States, it was undoubtedly present by the early 1970s and probably even earlier. By 1978, 4 percent of a large sample of gay and bisexual men in San Francisco were already HIV antibody positive ("Update" 1985). Overall HIV seroprevalence data in a study of pregnant women in New York City, the epicenter of AIDS in the United States, indicates that about 1.6 percent are positive. This is cause for grave concern. Yet, by comparison, a large sample of blood donors in Kigali, Rwanda in 1985 indicated that 17.5 percent were positive (Van de Perre, Kanyamupira et al. 1985). By 1986, the proportion rose to 24 percent (Anonymous 1986). Unpublished data indicate that in Bujumbura, Burundi, over 30 percent of a sample of blood donors were positive in early 1987 (Anonymous 1987).

The most fundamental question facing AIDS researchers in the area of international epidemiology is: Why is HIV infection spreading so rapidly among heterosexual men and women in central and east Africa, while so apparently slowly among nonintravenous (IV) drug-using heterosexual men and women in the United States? The quick pace of HIV spread among heterosexuals in central and east Africa closely parallels the rate of increase among gay and bisexual men and IV drug users in North America and western Europe. While studies in the United States have demonstrated high rates of seroconversion among steady partners of persons with AIDS, the proportion of all reported cases of AIDS which are known to be caused through heterosexual contact, excluding persons born in Haiti and other developing nations where HIV infection is common, is only 3.0 percent (Centers for Disease Control 1989).

In New York City, for example, most non-IV drug-using women with AIDS who have not had a blood transfusion became infected through unprotected sexual activity with a male IV drug user with AIDS (*New York City Monthly Surveillance Report,* 1989). For unknown reasons, very few women with AIDS in that city appear to have become infected through unprotected sexual activity with an HIV infected bisexual man. Except for the IV drug using route of transmission, then, why *is* HIV infection spreading more slowly into and through the general heterosexual population in the United States than in Rwanda?

The answer is probably multicausal, involving a complex interaction of parasitic, viral, and sociocultural cofactors. It is reasonably certain that HIV is the cause of AIDS. Peter Duesberg's (1987) claim that HIV is not the cause of AIDS has been brilliantly refuted in a review article by Kathleen McAuliff (1988). However, it is equally reasonably certain that HIV does not function within a biological vacuum, but is influenced by key cofactors.

Protozoal parasitic infections were first observed in a gay male in New York City in 1968. By the late 1970s, one study conducted in New York City by stool examination among a sample of completely asymptomatic gay and bisexual men indicated that nearly 40 percent were infected with intestinal parasites, especially

*Entamoeba histolytica* (which can cause amebiasis) and *Giardia lamblia* (which can cause giardiasis). Ethnographic data collected by this author suggests that the rise of protozoal infection in the gay communities of large U.S. cities during the 1970s correlates with an increase in anilingus (oral-anal activity) among gay and bisexual men. This increase is reflected, or perhaps was to some extent promoted by, a gradual increase in anilingus activity depicted in mostly U.S.-made all-male X-rated films from the late 1960s to the early 1980s.

By the late 1970s, special commercial laboratories designed exclusively for stool examination in primarily gay and bisexual men were set up in major U.S. cities for the diagnoses of these gastrointestinal parasites (Pearce 1983). There was a growing concern in the gay population of these diseases, and this concern apparently contributed to increasing caution in sexual activity with multiple partners among a subset of the gay population even before the herpes scare in the early 1980s and before AIDS was known and discussed.

Many intestinal parasites have been found to be immunosuppressive ("On Three Stages" 1986). A study conducted among a group of immunosuppressed cancer patients who were given a blood transfusion that was HIV contaminated, demonstrated that nine of ten surviving patients seroconverted to HIV infection—a higher rate than what would otherwise be expected in a healthy population with intact functioning immune systems (Anderson et al. 1986). It is possible that gay and bisexual men with symptomatic, or more commonly, asymptomatic protozoal infections are more likely to have weakened immune systems and are more susceptible to HIV infection upon exposure. Likewise, protozoal infections are very common throughout most of central and east Africa. In Rwanda, cryptosporidia are very common.

Microsporidia are minute protozoa, less than one-thousandth the diameter of an amoeba. They can only be diagnosed through intestinal biopsy, and there is no cure available. They were first diagnosed in the United States in a Haitian immigrant, and were recently diagnosed in six gay or bisexual men with AIDS. In sub-Saharan Africa, *Microspora* has been identified as a cause of malabsorption, resulting in a "wasting syndrome" (Cali 1988; Sprague and Vbavra 1976; Vivier 1975). Though four microsporidian genera have been identified in humans, only one (*Enterocytozoon bienusi*) seems to be repeatedly associated with symptomatic HIV infection (Cali and Owen 1989).

A Centers for Disease Control-sponsored research team will soon be looking at the possibility that heterosexuals in Africa and gay and bisexual men (as well as possibly IV drug users) in North America and Europe who are HIV infected and experience the "wasting syndrome" are doing so because they are co-infected with microsporidia. An effort will be made by the research team to develop a serological test for the diagnosis of microsporidia. A cure for these bacteria-like protozoa could probably be more readily developed than a cure for a retrovirus (Cali 1988).

*Microspora* have been found to be substantially immunosuppressive in fish, and may be immunosuppressive in humans as well. Accordingly, persons with microsporidia would be more likely to be immunocompromised and, therefore, to seroconvert if exposed to HIV, and asymptomatic HIV-infected persons who become infected with microsporidia would be more likely to rapidly develop weakened immunity and become symptomatic for AIDS.

Viruses may also play an important cofactor role in either enhancing the likelihood of HIV infection during exposure or promoting AIDS-related symptomatology in persons already HIV-infected. It is known that HIV-infected persons who continue to practice unprotected sex (Carne et al. 1987) or who continue to share unclean needles (Des Jarlais 1986) are more likely to rapidly develop the symptoms of AIDS than are HIV-infected persons who engage in safer sex practices or who stop sharing unclean needles. Cofactor viruses, such as cytomegalovirus (CMV), Epstein-Barr virus (EBV), and human T-cell leukemia virus type one (HTLV–1) may activate the T-cells of an HIV–1-infected person, stimulating the replication of HIV–1 virions, and hastening immunosuppression. An alternative view would suggest that immunosuppressive viruses, such as EBV and possibly the recently discovered human herpes virus, type six (HHV–6), may interact with HIV–1 to produce the deterioration of the immune system themselves. HHV–6 was discovered among AIDS patients in West Africa and Uganda, and surprisingly also among healthy blood donors in Great Britain, in 1987 (Downing et al. 1987; Tedder et al. 1987). Lusso et al. (1989) have recently concluded that HHV–6 "is a particularly suitable candidate as a cofactor in AIDS."

Epizootic diseases may also have relevance to the epidemiology of AIDS. The etiologic relationship between HIV–2 and simian immunodeficiency virus (SIV) in Old World monkeys is now clear, though HIV–1 is much more distantly related to both HIV–2 and SIV (Essex 1989). Also, an apparently nonpathogenic HIV-like virus has been found among Amazonian Indians in Brazil. It is possible that this may have occurred through contact with New World monkeys (Black 1987).

Jane Teas (1983) originally formulated the hypothesis that a new variant of African swine fever virus (ASFV) may be the etiologic agent of AIDS before it was known that HIV causes AIDS. ASFV is defined by some as an iridovirus (for example, Quintero et al. 1986), and by others as a pox virus (Carvalho and Rodrigues-Pousada 1986; Del Val et al. 1986). ASFV causes AIDS-like illness in pigs and goats (Wardley et al. 1983). The epidemiology of African Swine Fever (ASF) closely parallels the epidemiology of AIDS. ASF epidemics among pig populations most recently occurred in Zaire in 1971, in Haiti in 1978, in Rwanda in 1983, and elsewhere (Feldman 1986b; Wardley et al. 1983). ASF entered Malawi in 1981 from Zambia, a nation coincidentally which currently has a very high prevalence of AIDS cases (Haresnape et al. 1985).

Research conducted by John Beldekas et al. (1986) in the United States suggests that a sample of persons with AIDS may be infected with a mutated form of ASFV. Ten of 21 persons with AIDS, but only one of 16 controls, displayed a positive pattern for ASFV. An examination of 16 pigs in Belle Glades, Florida (a migrant worker community with an unusually high rate of persons with AIDS) did not reveal ASFV among them, however (Feorino et al. 1986). In what has been described as an unrelated action, the U.S. government began irradiating all pork sold in the United States a few months after this study.

In Rwanda, ASF entered in the south-central part of the country near Butare. Half of the nation's pig population died in a matter of months. Those that survived have developed a chronic infection without illness (Feldman 1986b). A study of female prostitutes in Butare in 1984 yielded an 82 percent rate of HIV symptomatic infection (Van de Perre, Clumeck et al. 1985). One hospitalized informant with AIDS in Kigali reported to this author in 1985 that ingesting goat urine is a common therapeutic treatment administered by traditional healers in urban and rural Rwanda. In his particular case, he ingested goat urine after he first began to develop HIV-related symptoms, but discontinued the treatment because it made him feel much worse. He did not ingest goat urine at any time before developing the symptoms.

William Hess (1987) of the U.S. Department of Agriculture Plum Island facility, who has worked extensively in ASFV research, expressed to this author his view that data are insufficient from an epidemiologic perspective to rule out a possible link between ASF and AIDS. Though ASFV and HIV are very different kinds of viruses (Martins and Lawman 1986; Temin 1987), the possibility that a variant of ASFV may play a contributory role as a cofactor in enhancing HIV infectivity and/or disease progress has not yet been thoroughly investigated. Recently, Lo et al. (1989) found that four silvered-leaf monkeys, inoculated with a virus-like infectious agent derived from cells from an AIDS patient, showed wasting and died within nine months. It is not known whether the virus-like infectious agent is related to ASFV. Ethnographic analyses and medical evaluations should be conducted among pig farmers and goat herders in sub-Saharan Africa.

Sociocultural variables may play a crucial role in enhancing or inhibiting HIV and AIDS. Sexual behavior differences may provide several excellent examples. With few exceptions, such as the Mbuti of Zaire, sexual activity is prohibited during menstruation in rural central and east Africa. However, in many African cities, including Kigali, the prohibition against sex during menstruation is frequently no longer followed (Taylor 1987). It is likely that a menstruating woman engaging in sexual intercourse would more readily transmit HIV to her partner, or become HIV infected by her partner. Systematic research is needed to compare sexual activity during menstruation in rural versus urban Africa, in the United States, and in traditional African cultures where sex during menstruation had never been prohibited.

Rates of heterosexual activity in parts of Africa compared to the United States have been suggested by some as an explanation for higher HIV seroprevalence in Africa. However, in Rwanda, for example, the culture has been fairly sexually restrictive concerning premarital sex for women (Werner 1990). Only a generation ago, unwed mothers were drowned in rivers as punishment (see Taylor,

Chapter 5, this volume). Today, there is greater permissiveness, but for women, Rwandan premarital sexual morality is still more restrictive than contemporary urban American mores would allow. Men tend to marry fairly late, with a mean age of 28.4 years in Kigali. Sexual activity with prostitutes is common for men especially in their late twenties before marriage in Kigali (Carael et al. 1985).

Extramarital relations for both men and women in Rwanda were always more open (Maquet 1961). Nevertheless, a major sweep of female prostitutes occurred in the early 1980s in Rwanda (unrelated to the AIDS issue) where oppressive measures were taken, imprisoning most prostitutes in "re-education" camps (Taylor 1987). Eighteen percent of all households in Rwanda remain polygynous (Carael et al. 1985). In Kinshasa, Zaire, married men often have sexual relations with unmarried younger women (Ryder 1988). In general, there does not appear to be a correlation between lower HIV seroprevalence and greater sexual restrictiveness cross-culturally in Africa. Within urban central and east African cities, though, female prostitutes and their male clients are most likely to be HIV infected and to have AIDS (Kreiss et al. 1986).

In Rwanda, there is no recreational IV drug use. However, a recreational hallucinogenic drug named "chanvre" (urumogi in Kinyarwanda) is smoked or drunk by teenagers and sexually active persons in their twenties in Kigali. It was formerly used only by the Twa (a pygmy population) in their villages. Many recreational drugs have been found to be immunocompromising, and it would be useful to conduct research to determine if this is valid for "chanvre," in order to predict a possible role for the drug in enhancing HIV infectivity.

Untreated sexually transmissible diseases are generally common throughout sub-Saharan Africa and include (besides AIDS) syphilis, gonorrhea, herpes, hepatitis B, chancroid, lymphogranuloma venereum, and others. One informant with AIDS in Rwanda said that he often had sex with female prostitutes during his herpes outbreaks. Even though it was admittedly painful, he did not wish to forego the pleasure of having sex. Obviously, open penile lesions would promote HIV infectivity. It is also likely that, since AIDS reactivates latent cases of syphilis, symptoms of tertiary syphilis are quite common in Rwanda where this disease is so prevalent.

In Rwanda, anti-HIV surveillance indicates that there is a tenfold greater rate of prevalence in Kigali than in some rural villages (Lepage et al. 1985). Except for villages in southwestern Uganda, northwestern Tanzania, and now northern Rwanda (near the Ugandan border), AIDS is primarily an urban disease in Africa. This is perhaps one of the most baffling questions facing anthropologists who will work in the area of AIDS in Africa. With such continual movement of people between the cities, towns, and villages, why is not the distribution of HIV–1 infection among sexually active men and women, their partners, and their children more equal regardless of the location? The general dichotomy between high seroprevalence in urban Africa and low seroprevalence in rural Africa does not make sense. Moreover, in parts of rural Africa where traditional practices such as ritual, aesthetic, and therapeutic scarification, as well as blood-brotherhood practices and group male circumcision activities should still occur, HIV-1 transmission would be further enhanced. In one rural region of Zaire, however, the rate of HIV seroprevalence inexplicably remained stable at the 0.8 percent level from 1976 to 1986 (Nzilambi et al. 1988), even though it is located along a busy commercial waterway.

In Rwanda, mandatory identity cards attempt to control rural-urban migration within the small country. Persons found in Kigali without a job, originating from outside the city, are imprisoned for a month and returned to their village. But still they come. Kigali has grown from a population of 5,000 in 1960 to over 250,000 today.

To summarize, the key epidemiologic questions of AIDS have not yet been answered. It will require anthropological research and insights, working in cooperation with epidemiologists, veterinary scientists, clinicians, parasitologists, virologists, and immunologists, to unlock this highly complex puzzle. It is not being maintained here that the sexually active non-IV drug using heterosexual population in the United States has little to worry about. Quite the contrary. Articles in popular magazines asserting that condoms are not necessary for this population (see, for example, Gould 1988) will tragically cause the unnecessary deaths of many women. The inhibiting cofactors among non-IV drug using heterosexuals in the United States and other developed nations will only slow the spread of AIDS. They will not stop it. It appears inevitable that if risk reduction interventions are not carried out, non-IV drug using heterosexual spread of the virus in North America and Europe may eventually become the most prevalent form, especially in the inner cities.

To the extent that cofactors may alter the likelihood of HIV infection and the progression of symptomatology, cofactor research is important in elucidating these patterns for possible therapeutic applications. It may prove easier to manipulate, modify, or eliminate biological and sociocultural cofactors than to attack HIV and AIDS directly.

## NOTE

This chapter is based in part on research conducted in Rwanda in 1985. I wish to thank the AIDS Medical Foundation for their generous support, and Dr. Mathilde Krim for her strong encouragement. I would like to thank Dr. Francis P. Conant, Dr. Emilio Mantero-Atienza, and Dr. Priscilla Reining for their comments on this paper. I would also like to thank Dr. Ann Cali, Dr. Don C. Des Jarlais, Dr. Francis Black, and Dr. Christopher Taylor in providing information for this paper. An earlier draft of this paper was read at the American Association for the Advancement of Science meeting in Boston in February 1988.

## REFERENCES

Anderson, K.C., et al. (1986). "Transfusion-acquired human immunodeficiency virus infection among immunocompromised persons." *Annals of Internal Medicine* 105:519–27.

Anonymous. (1986). Personal communication.

Anonymous. (1987). Personal communication.

Beldekas, John; Jane Teas; and James R. Herbert. (1986). "African swine fever virus and AIDS." *Lancet* 1 (8480):564–65.

Black, Francis. (1987). Personal communication.

Cali, Ann. (1988). Personal communication.

Cali, Ann, and R.L. Owen. (1989). "Microsporidiosia and ARC." Fifth International Conference on AIDS, Montreal, June.

Carael, Michael; P. Van de Perre; E. Akingeneye et al. (1985). "Socio-cultural factors in relation to HTLV-III/LAV transmission in urban areas in central Africa." International Conference on African AIDS, Brussels, November.

Carne, C.A., et al. (1987). "Prevalence of antibodies to human immunodeficiency virus, gonorrhoea rates, and changed sexual behavior in homosexual men in London." *Lancet* 1(8534):656–58.

Carvalho, Z.G., and C. Rodrigues-Pousada. (1986). "African swine fever virus gene expression in infected vero cells." *Journal of General Virology* 67:1343–50.

Centers for Disease Control. (1989). *HIV/AIDS Surveillance,* June.

Clumeck, Nathan; J. Sonnet; H. Taelman; F. Mascart-Lemone; M. deBruyere et al. (1984). "Acquired immunodeficiency syndrome in African patients." *New England Journal of Medicine* 310(8):492–97.

Del Val, M.; J.L. Carrascosa; and E. Vinuela. (1986). "Glycosylated components of African swine fever virus particles." *Virology* 152:39–49.

Des Jarlais, Don C. (1986). Personal communication.

Downing, R.G., et al. (1987). "Isolation of human lymphotropic herpesvirus from Uganda." *Lancet* 2(8555):390.

Duesberg, Peter H. (1987). "Retroviruses as carcinogens and pathogens: expectations and reality." *Cancer Research* 47:1199–1220, March 1.

Essex, M. (1989). "The origins of human retroviruses." Paper read at the Fifth International Conference on AIDS, Montreal, June.

Feldman, Douglas A. (1986a). "Anthropology, AIDS, and Africa." *Medical Anthropology Quarterly* 17 (2):38–40.

———. (1986b). "An African swine fever link with AIDS?" (letter) *New York Times,* July 31.

———. (1989). "A household survey for suspected AIDS-related complex in Rwanda." *Medical Anthropology.*

Feldman, Douglas A.; Samuel Friedman; and Don Des Jarlais. (1987). "Public awareness of AIDS in Rwanda." *Social Science and Medicine* 24(2):97–100.

Feldman, Douglas A., and Christopher Taylor (forthcoming). "Blood, sex and AIDS in Rwanda."

Feorino, P.; G. Schable; G. Schachetman et al. (1986). "AIDS and African swine fever virus." *Lancet* 2 (8510):815, October 4.

Gould, R.E. (1988). "Reassuring news about AIDS: A doctor tells why you may not be at risk." *Cosmopolitan* 204:146, January.

Haresnape, J.M.; S.A.M. Lungu; and F.D. Mamu. (1985). "A four-year survey of African swine fever in Malawi." *Journal of Hygiene* 95:309–23.

Hess, William. (1987). Personal communication.

Kanki, P.J., et al. (1985). "Serological identification and characterization of a macaque

T-lymphotropic retrovirus closely related to HTLV-III." *Science* 228(4704):1199–1201.

Kreiss, J.K., et al. (1986). "AIDS virus infection in Nairobi prostitutes: Spread of the epidemic to East Africa." *New England Journal of Medicine* 314(7):414–18.

Lepage, Philippe; P. Van de Perre; C. Van Goethem et al. (1985). "HTLV-III/LAV infected children and their families." International Conference on African AIDS, Brussels, November.

Lepage, Philippe; P. Van de Perre; M. Carael; and J.P. Butzler. (1986). "Are medical injections a risk factor for HIV infection in children?" *Lancet* 2(8515):1103–4.

Lo, S.-C.; R.Y.-H. Wang; P.B. Newton III; N.-Y.Yang; M.A. Sonoda; and J.W.-K. Shih. (1989). "Fatal infection of silvered leaf monkeys with a virus-like infectious agent (VLIA) derived from a patient with AIDS." *Amer. Jour. Trop. Med. Hyg.* 40(4):399–409.

Lusso, P., et al. 1989. "Human herpesvirus 6 (HHV–6) as a potential cofactor in AIDS." Poster at the Fifth International Conference on AIDS, Montreal, June.

Maquet, J.J.P. (1961). *The Premise of Inequality in Ruanda: A Study of Political Relations in a Central African Kingdom.* London: Oxford University Press.

Martins, C.V., and M.J.P. Lawman. (1986). "African swine fever and AIDS." *Lancet* 1 (8496):1504–5, June 28.

McAuliffe, Kathleen. (1988). "The Etiology of AIDS: A report on the AmFAR Scientific Forum, Washington, D.C., April 9, 1988." *AIDS Targeted Information Newsletter* 2(5):1–3, May.

Nahmias, Andre; J. Weiss; X. Yao et al. (1986). "Evidence for human infection with an HTLV-III/LAV-like virus in central Africa, 1959." *Lancet* 1(8492):1279–80.

*New York City Monthly Surveillance Report.* (1989). New York City Department of Health, May.

Nzilambi, N.; K.M. de Cock; D.N. Forthal et al. (1988). "The prevalence of infection with human immunodeficiency virus over a 10-year period in rural Zaire." *New England Journal of Medicine* 318:276–79.

"On three stages of amoebic research." (1986). *Lancet* 2(8516):1133–34.

Pearce, R.B. (1983). "Intestinal protozoal infections and AIDS." *Lancet* 2:51.

Quintero, J.C.,; R.D. Wesley; T.C. Whyard; D. Gregg; and C.A. Mebus (1986). "In vitro and in vivo association of African swine fever virus with swine erythrocytes." *Am. J. Vet. Res.* 47(5):1125–31, May.

Ryder, R. (1988). "Heterosexual and perinatal transmission of HIV infection." American Association for the Advancement of Sciences meeting, Boston, February.

Sprague, V., and J. Vbavra (1976). "Biology of the microsporidia." In L.A., Bulla and T.C. Cheng, (eds.), *Comparative Pathobiology*, pp. 1–371. Plenum Press: New York.

Taylor, Christopher. (1987). Personal communication.

Teas, Jane. (1983). "Could AIDS agent be a new variant of African Swine Fever Virus?" *Lancet* 1(8330):923, April 23.

Tedder, R.S., et al. (1987). "A novel lymphotropic herpesvirus." *Lancet* 2(8555):390–92.

Temin, Howard. (1987). Personal communication.

"Update: acquired immunodeficiency syndrome in the San Francisco cohort study, 1978–1985." 1985. *MMWR* 32(38):573–75.

Van de Perre, P.; N. Clumeck; M. Carael; E. Nzabihimana; M. Robert-Guroff; P. DeMol;

R. Freyens; J.P. Butzler; R.C. Gallo; and J.B. Kanyamupira. (1985). "Female prostitutes: A risk group for infection with human T-cell lymphotropic virus type III." *Lancet* 2(8454):524–26.

Van de Perre, P.; J. B. Kanyamupira; M. Carael et al. (1985). "HTLV-III/LAV infection in central Africa." International Conference on African AIDS, Brussels, November.

Van de Perre, P., et al. (1984). "Acquired immunodeficiency syndrome in Rwanda." *Lancet* 2(8394):62–65.

Vivier, E. (1975). "The microsporidia of the Protozoa." *Protistologica* 11:345–61.

Wardley, R.C.; C. de M. Andrade; D.N. Black et al. (1983). "African swine fever virus: brief review." *Archives of Virology* 76(2):73–90.

Werner, Dennis. (1990). *Human Sexuality around the World.* New Haven: HRAF Press.

# Chapter Five

## AIDS and the Pathogenesis of Metaphor

Christopher C. Taylor

As AIDS continues to spread its way from one part of the world to another and from one sector of the U.S. population to another, it is becoming increasingly clear that societies are being forced to come to grips with two aspects of AIDS pathology, one which is directed toward AIDS the "disease" and another which is oriented toward AIDS the "illness." This disease/illness distinction (Kleinman, Eisenberg & Good, 1978: 251–52) differentiates between "disease," the biological and psychophysiological malfunctions occasioned by sickness,[1] and "illness," the manner in which a specific sickness is experienced by the sufferer (1978: 251–52) and culturally labeled, explained, and valued (Kleinman, 1980: 72). While biomedical practitioners generally concern themselves almost exclusively with the "disease" component of AIDS, it is apparent that for sufferers and society the "illness" component of AIDS is also important. AIDS as "illness" incorporates judgments about its meaning for sufferers and society, judgments that are culturally specific and receive expression through the medium of metaphor.

For example, we know that HIV suppresses the immune system, that in its later stages it invites "opportunistic infections," and that AIDS is almost always fatal; these are characteristics of the "disease," AIDS. However, many Americans fear and detest AIDS more for its perceived association with a "debauched" life-style, most notably, homosexuality and intravenous drug use, than for any direct health threat to themselves. The moral judgments leveled against gay men and IV drug users by certain segments of the American population have become part of AIDS as "illness," part of AIDS as a "social construct" (cf. Berger & Luckman, 1967). This construct, I maintain, has influenced the response that American health authorities have taken against AIDS as much as, if not more than, scientific thinking about the "disease" component of AIDS.

Furthermore, the atmosphere of moral opprobrium evoked by AIDS has become as potentially harmful to society as the "disease" AIDS is to persons with AIDS. It is in this sense that AIDS has given rise to another pathogenic process, the production of socially destructive "illness" metaphors. Many people see AIDS as the sign of divine wrath directed against a society, in recapitulation of Sodom and Gomorrah, which has grown too permissive. From this perspective AIDS can only be cast out when the moral evils of society have been scourged and purified.

Although societies differ in the moral judgments they make about specific sicknesses and about the experience of sickness in general, all share a tendency to use sickness as a figure or metaphor. Susan Sontag (1977) laments this tendency and calls for a view of sickness that eliminates metaphoric thinking. Using a profusion of literary examples, Sontag shows that people afflicted with tuberculosis (TB) in the nineteenth century tended to be portrayed as persons who became ill because of their rarefied artistic and erotic sensibilities. In other instances, writers depicted TB sufferers as the victims of a poverty-stricken or otherwise harsh environment (Sontag, 1977: 15). In either case tuberculosis ennobled the sufferer, lifting him or her above the common plane of ordinary humanity to a semi-mystical locus between life and death. Placing TB sanitariums in the mountains was indicative perhaps, of the nineteenth-century tendency to socially situate TB sufferers closer to heaven than to earth. Thomas Mann's *The Magic Mountain* (1924), for example, with its curious mixture of spiritual striving and social decadence seems to follow in this mode.

The twentieth-century person with cancer on the other hand, has received rather bad press, for he is portrayed as repressed, self-loathing, and emotionally inert (Sontag, 1978: 53). He is someone whose refusal to deal with his innermost feelings has left him prone to attack by destructive forces within his own body. Sontag cites the maverick psychoanalyst, Wilhelm Reich, as one of the chief proponents of this negative stereotype, for he attributed cancer to "emotional resignation" and "bio-energetic shrinking" (Sontag, 1977: 23). Since Sontag suffered from cancer herself, as well as from its characterization, she feels that the metaphors we create about disease are often as afflicting as the diseases themselves. One might think, therefore, that Sontag is advocating a "scientific," that is, value-free view of sickness, but many of the culprits in her story are medical scientists themselves. What seem like "facts" to these scientists, often turn out to be merely the value judgments about a disease which were in vogue at a particular social and historical juncture.

What Sontag advocates, however, is probably unrealizable; it is doubtful that there will ever be a completely metaphor-free view of all sicknesses, or in Kleinman's terms, "disease" without "illness." While certain sicknesses do not engender illness metaphors because of their innocuousness, sicknesses that are contagious, life-threatening, characterized by bizarre or debilitating symptoms, or associated with abnormal behavior are likely to give rise to imagery embodying positive or negative sociomoral judgments. Moreover, these judgments are further reinforced when the sickness manifests a propensity to afflict members of society who are already marginalized for reasons of ethnicity, life-style, or socioeconomic status.

Western culture abounds with historical examples of illness metaphors which, in my opinion, have served as models for those associated with AIDS today. Leprosy, for example, was clearly conceptualized according to notions of ritual purity. Biblical references to the "cleansing" of lepers illustrate this point, supporting Douglas's thesis (1966) that persons or things perceived to be "out of place" or classificatorily ambiguous tend to be treated as socially dangerous. In the Middle Ages, for example, many communities forced their lepers to live apart from the healthy. At the first symptoms of affliction, lepers underwent a "rite de passage"—a funeral mass—to mark their "death" (Gaignebet, 1974: 66–68). While lying in a coffin, the leper was read a list of the rules that would govern his future interaction with healthy people: prohibition against touching anything unless this was done with a stick, prohibition against approaching wells and springs, prohibition against speaking except when the wind was blowing in one's face (Gaignebet, 1974: 67). Once this mass was celebrated, the person left his home and family to live in a community with other lepers.

Once in this community, lepers could continue their lives unmolested only if they accepted the "liminal" existence (Turner, 1969) combining biological life and social death, which healthy society allotted them. Economically, leper communities were subjected to occupational marginalization. They gained their livelihood by exercising ritually "dangerous" activities such as rope-making (Gaignebet, 1974: 65–86). Rope-making was "dangerous," because ropes were "liminal;" they traversed boundaries, they linked disparate realms of space, and in hanging condemned prisoners, they mediated the passage between life and death. Furthermore, medieval ropes were manufactured from hemp (*Cannabis sativa*). The discarded portions of the plant were burnt and undoubtedly the intoxicating fumes of the marijuana were inhaled (Gaignebet, 1974: 66). This conjunction of sickness, social marginality, and drug-induced pleasure was perhaps the first instance in Western epidemiologic history of themes foreshadowing our present imagery of AIDS.

Closer to AIDS because of its association with sexuality, syphilis has also been colorfully painted by the metaphoric brush. Fracastoro, the famed Italian Renaissance poet who wrote in Latin (cf. Eatough, 1984), gave the disease its name, attributing its origin to the hubris of a young shepherd named Syphilis, who dared to venerate his earthly king, Alcithous, above the Sun God, Apollo. Angered, Apollo afflicted the shepherd with the pestilence that came to bear his name. Cure came only after Syphilis expiated his fault through sacrifice (Eatough, 1984: 21). Fracastoro lived during a time of tremendous upheaval, the sixteenth century—an age of plagues, religious wars, voyages of discovery, and the expansion of mercantile capitalism (cf. Wallerstein, 1976). In explicitly comparing the contraction of syphilis to the breach of a ritual injunction, Fracastoro reflected an attitude that was quite widespread, for syphilis had begun to replace leprosy as a focus of religious concern (Eatough, 1984: 4). Furthermore, evidence from his time demonstrates that his Spanish contemporaries were using the specter of syphilis as a hegemonic tool to justify their conquest of the New World on the grounds that Native Americans were inferior beings, "pagans" and originators of the syphilitic plague (Eatough, 1984: 13). Syphilis was also used to reinforce xenophobic stereotypes. Italians called syphilis the "Spanish disease," French called it the "Neapolitan disease," English called it the "French disease," and Russians, the "Polish disease" (Barnouw & Clark, 1955: 4).

The most recent of the "great plagues," AIDS follows a pattern that is similar to those which preceded it. Perhaps this explains the hypothesis (Coulter, 1987) which places *Treponema pallidum*—the spirochete that causes syphilis—at the basis of the AIDS pandemic. Furthermore, this hypothesis relegates what is widely believed to be the virus that causes AIDS, HIV–1, to the status of a mere cofactor (Coulter, 1987: 66). This hypothesis has not, however, met with wide approval. One might further wonder if the resemblance between the "illness" of syphilis and the "illness" of AIDS has influenced this tendency of linking the two diseases. After all, scientists are not as free of metaphoric thinking as believers in science would like to have it.

Moreover, whether or not medical scientists intend this result, many of their research findings that receive attention in the press. become input which contributes to the metaphoric elaboration of AIDS. Consider, for example, the question of geographical origin. In Rwanda, where I did field research on traditional medicine for 21 months, people believe that AIDS originated with gay men and IV drug users in the United States and Europe, and then spread to Rwanda with tourists. In the United States, on the other hand, we usually hear that AIDS has an African origin. Some theories trace the migration of the disease in this way: green monkeys transmitted the virus to Africans. Africans then gave the disease to Haitians working in Zaire and/or Cuban soldiers in Angola, who brought it back to the Caribbean. American gay men vacationing in Haiti brought the disease from the Caribbean to urban centers in the United States, where it was picked up by IV drug users. From there it began to spread to the white heterosexual population.

Although a great deal of research remains to be done to confirm or deny the validity of these hypotheses concerning the geographic trajectory of AIDS (though it is certain now that African green monkeys are not the source of AIDS), my point does not concern their truth value. Instead what interests me about these hypotheses is, first of all, their potential to be used metaphorically, and second, their capacity to justify xenophobic stereotypes in the popular imagination.

Let us take the idea that AIDS originated with monkeys, spread to sub-Saharan Africans, then moved on to gay men and IV drug users, before finding its way into heterosexual white society. There is an evolutionist cast to this scenario, something which resembles the eighteenth- and nineteenth-century belief in the "great chain of being" (cf. Lovejoy, 1933). This belief, it should be recalled, maintained that there was a gradual rise of beings from the least exalted to the most divine. Humankind, though beneath the angels, was superior to all other forms of biological life. In subsequent versions of the "great chain of being" idea, human races were arranged hierarchically according to their proximity or distance from divinity. It is not surprising that the originators of these ideas, who were white European males, believed that the highest rung of human evolution had been attained by male members of white European society. (Precursors to these notions, incidentally, can already be discerned in the sixteenth-century view of syphilis.) Added to this evolutionist idea, there was a diffusionist one: The absurd belief that everything progressive came from Europe and everything atavistic came from elsewhere.

One of the most deleterious results of these ideas was that they tended to become reified in nineteenth-century "science." The nascent study of anthropology, for example, reflected European lay society's prejudices and self-satisfaction (cf. Gould, 1981). Skulls from various races were measured and compared according to the theory that intercranial volume reflected intelligence. Not surprisingly, these researchers found in "objective reality," what they had already formulated in their own minds before the first skull was measured—Caucasians had the largest skull volume while Africans had the smallest (Gould, 1981: 66). Although the work of these "scientists" has since been refuted, it must be noted that a similar theory has reemerged with the practice of testing for "intelligence quotient" or I.Q. As recently as 1979, Arthur Jensen has defended an hereditarian theory of I.Q. that essentially recapitulates the "great chain of being" idea (Gould, 1981: 317). Jensen claims that the "intelligence" of all animal life can be quantified and assigned a numerical value (Gould 1981: 317). Not surprisingly, he situates black people on one of the lowest rungs of humankind. Africa has remained the "Dark Continent" in too many minds, a focus for fear, as well as for romantic projection.

My question then becomes: Is the origin story of AIDS, as it is construed in the United States, giving rise to metaphors that are inspired by and thus resemble the "great chain of being" idea? Is AIDS ontogeny recapitulating a false phylogeny? By placing lower primates at the beginning of the infectious chain, white male heterosexuals at the end of the chain, and black people, Hispanics, gay men, and IV drug users at intermediate points along it, aren't we running the risk of pointing the finger of responsibility for AIDS in the direction of people whom heterosexual white society perceives to be less highly evolved than itself? There is strong evidence that this is indeed the case, and that the "illness" perception of AIDS in the United States has contributed to the propagation of the "disease" through the failure to take it seriously.

Randy Shilts (1988) demonstrates that as long as white, middle-class, heterosexual Americans did not feel threatened by AIDS, there was little impetus on the part of politicians and public health authorities (with a few notable exceptions) to come to grips with the problem. To some observers, this indifference was conspicuous. In 1981, for example, commentator Frank Gifford wondered why, in the face of evidence that AIDS was spreading rapidly, no one was paying any attention to it (Shilts, 1988: 110). Later in April, 1982, Congressman Waxman made the cogent observation (1988: 143–44) that AIDS, unlike "Legionnaire's Disease," struck the socially unacceptable and was thus being ignored by the political establishment. The amounts of money spent on disease research in the United States during the first years of the AIDS epidemic are quite telling. While the National Institutes of Health spent an average of $34,841 in 1981 for each person who died of "Legionnaire's Disease," only $3,225 was spent by the same organization in 1981 for each person who died of AIDS, and only $8,991 in 1982 (Shilts 1988: 186). Clearly the hierarchy of national health priorities during this time tended to reflect "illness" perceptions.

Furthermore, many of the most inflammatory statements concerning AIDS emanated from persons in the center of the public eye. On May 24, 1983, columnist Patrick Buchanan, formerly director of White House communications, commented: "The poor homosexuals—they have declared war upon nature, and now nature is exacting an awful retribution" (Shilts, 1988: 311). Two months later, "Moral Majority" leader Jerry Falwell echoed these sentiments with the observation that, "When you violate moral, health, and hygiene laws, you reap the whirlwind. You cannot shake your fist in God's face and get by with it" (Shilts, 1988: 347). The comments of these two men are not just noteworthy for their obvious insensitivity, what is also of interest is the direct relationship of these statements to illness metaphors employed in the Middle Ages and the sixteenth century. Although some elements of white heterosexual American society can still imagine themselves at the evolutionary pinnacle of the "great chain of being," the attitudes of its spokespersons with regard to sickness have not really advanced much in the past four centuries.

## AIDS AS "ILLNESS" IN RWANDA

It is interesting to compare our notions about AIDS with those prevalent in Rwanda. According to our ideas, Rwanda is situated very close to the geographical epicenter of the AIDS pandemic. But Rwandans, as I indicated earlier, see the disease as being of American and European origin and as having originated among gay men and IV drug users. While in Rwanda, I found a poster at the National University of Rwanda in Butare intended to warn students about AIDS. I was surprised, however, that the two figures in the poster, a man clad only in his underpants and a fully nude woman, did not have black features. While the artist may not have intended the poster to suggest this, the viewer might very well understand that AIDS is primarily a white disease. Another interesting aspect about this poster was that the woman was chasing the man and that it was the woman who was portrayed as infected. The poster was entitled, "Twilinde SIDA," meaning, "Let's guard against AIDS!" The woman in the drawing was depicted as saying, "Come, let me give it to you," while the man running away from her replies, "Oh, no! You won't infect me with AIDS!"

It would seem from this poster that the artist was attributing responsibility for the spread of AIDS in Rwanda first to Europeans and Americans, and second, to women. This second aspect, relating to women, is of interest for it reflects the ambivalence of Rwandan cultural attitudes toward female sexuality. While Rwandan culture has always promoted healthy female sexuality, females were also, in former times, very closely surveyed. The reason for this was that female sexuality, when left to its own devices, was perceived as uncontrollable. There were very stringent measures of repression. Young women who became pregnant out of wedlock could be hurled from cliffs, thrown into rivers, or brought to islands in the middle of Lake Kivu and abandoned there. In some regions of Rwanda, I was told, these measures persisted until the early 1950s.

But it was also part of Rwandan cultural practices and values that young girls develop their sexuality in preparation for marriage. Pubescent and prepubescent girls in former times, and to some extent today, practiced *gukuna imishino na rugongo* (manual manipulation of labia majora and the clitoris to elongate them). Enlarged female genitalia were said to be preferred by men and, furthermore, they were thought to facilitate female orgasm. This was important, for, as traditional healers told me, conception is most likely to occur after both partners have had orgasm. The mothers of young girls encouraged their daughters to engage in *gukuna* and would sometimes ask to see their genitalia to verify this. To accomplish *gukuna*, young girls would go off to a secluded spot on the hillside and would be instructed in the practice by older adolescent girls. Sometimes a girl would insert her finger into a companion's vagina and then instruct her in how to move her pelvis in order to arrive at orgasm easily. In elongating their genitalia, however, Rwandan girls symbolically ran the risk of "phallicizing" themselves, and thus usurping a male perogative. There was a danger of their developing overly assertive sexuality. This theme repeatedly surfaces in Rwandan myth and legend.

Consider the following traditional Rwandan legend:

The wife that Gihanga had brought back from Burundi (south of Rwanda) became pregnant in her turn. During her pregnancy, a quarrel broke out by Gihanga. Nyiraru-cyaba, the eldest daughter of Gihanga, mortally wounded the Rundi wife by striking her in the stomach with a boar spear and she died, but the child she was bearing managed to escape safe and sound, although born prematurely. Gihanga named him Gafomo. [Gafomo: the "product of a Caesarean," cf. Smith, 1975: 286.] Nyirarucyaba fled and took refuge in the forest. There she was welcomed by a certain Kazigaba [an ancestor of the Zigaba clan]. She married him and they had children. One day, though, she learned that her father was very ill and she became sad.

Just then she saw cows emerging from the lake. One of the beasts came over and gave birth in front of her doorway. Then the calf became entangled in forest vines. Though its mother stayed with it, the other cattle began making their way back to the lake. Nyirarucyaba made a clay pot and went to milk the cow. Noticing that the milk had a pleasant taste, she bought the calf close to the entry of the hut and tethered it there. The cow followed.

Then Nyirarucyaba sent some of the milk she had discovered to her father through the intermediary of her mother. Gihanga, pleasantly surprised, had his daughter brought to him and gave her his forgiveness.

Nyirarucyaba brought other jugs with her. The milk cured Gihanga of his illness. Then he demanded that his son-in-law send him the cow. The son-in-law refused, so Gihanga grew angry. Finally, Nyirarucyaba brought the animal herself.

Then, once again, the wild cattle began to emerge from the lake, so Gihanga decided to take possession of them. But Gafomo, who had perched on top of a tree, screamed out in fright when he saw the immense herd. The cattle ran back to take refuge in the lake and it closed in on them. The narrator concludes: "Only a few cows remain. These are the ones that Rwandans have raised; if cattle had come in greater numbers, no man would be the ruler of another." (Cited in L. de Heusch, 1982: 52. Translation by this author.)

This myth is interesting for several reasons, but I will only consider the theme that directly concerns female roles and female sexuality. First of all, Rwandan woman are often symbolically equated to cattle because cows are exchanged for wives in bridewealth transactions. Furthermore, both women and cows are related to liquids because both produce milk, a white fluid, which in some mythico-ritual contexts is depicted as an analog to male semen (cf. Taylor, 1988).

This story shows the aquatic origin of cattle. Cattle in the myth are not simply metaphorically related to liquids, they are portrayed essentially as part of a liquid, in this case, the terrestrial waters of a lake. This association is more complex, though, than the simple observation that cattle produce milk and thus have an obvious connection to liquids. In bridewealth transactions, cattle and women "flow" in opposing "streams" in exchange for one another. Notice that a bridewealth exchange involving cattle takes place in this legend, as Gihanga demands that his son-in-law, Kazigaba, send him a cow. Kazigaba, however, refuses to send Gihanga a cow and finally, Nyirarucyaba must bring him the cow herself.

Nyirarucyaba acts the part of an overly phallicized woman in several ways in this legend. For example, notice that Nyirarucyaba ignores the taboo that prevents men and women from employing objects belonging to the other sex. A man must never handle the large wooden spoon that Rwandan women use to stir cooking food and a woman must never carry or use metal objects associated with hunting (Smith, 1979: p.30). Nyirarucyaba ignores this taboo by seizing a boar spear and killing her stepmother by slicing open her uterus. This action is the precipitant cause of the hapless Gafomo's birth. Nyirarucyaba, in usurping the powers of a "phallus" (the boar spear), is the immediate cause of a tragic being's birth, Gafomo, whose cry will eventually cause cattle to rush back into the lake.

Nyirarucyaba is thus the ultimate cause of the impeded flow of milk upon the earth. Milk, a white substance, is symbolically analogous to semen. Nyirarucyaba unwittingly deprives the world of a white fertility fluid by illegitimately assuming a male role. By "flowing" in the wrong direction, toward masculinity instead of femininity, Nyirarucyaba makes the cows "flow" the wrong way as well, that is, back into the lake instead of out of the lake. This observation is reinforced by Nyirarucyaba's role in bringing the cow that her father Gihanga has demanded of her husband, Kazigaba. Again Nyirarucyaba is assuming a male role— women do not act as their own agents nor as transactors in bridewealth exchange. Men exchange women; women do not exchange themselves. The same idea is illustrated in another Rwandan taboo analyzed by Smith (1979: 28). This taboo states that unmarried girls must not use cattle paths when walking over the hillsides. As Smith points out, this is because the exchange destinies of women and cattle are opposed. Women flow in one direction, cattle flow in the opposite direction. Both are objects of exchange and never its agents.

Today, the specter of Nyirarucyaba, the overly assertive or "phallicized" Rwandan female, continues to loom large in spite of the fact that the practice of *gukuna* is much less widely followed, due to the influence of Catholicism. Moreover, the severe measures of repression against premaritally pregnant girls have disappeared entirely (though abortion is severely punished). Many of the ambivalent attitudes associated with female sexuality, though, linger on. Women, especially in urban centers, enjoy greater freedom, but the belief persists that women should follow a stricter code of sexual conduct than men. In the spring and early summer of 1983, this attitude surfaced when hundreds of single, urban Rwandan women were rounded up, charged with "vagabondage," and placed in re-education camps. Although many of these women were indeed prostitutes, a much greater number were legally employed and guilty of nothing more than consorting with European men socially.

The French newspaper, *Libération,* commented sardonically upon this in an article entitled, "Touche pas à l'homme blanc," ("Don't touch the white man"). According to Rwandan men that I spoke with regarding these measures of repression, a few highly placed government ministers feared that the sexual mores of Rwandan women who had European fiancés or boyfriends could be corrupted. They might become prostitutes or take up European sexual practices such as fellatio, cunnilingus, and anal intercourse. Rwandan women thus continue to be regarded through the scrutinizing eyes of a male-centered society and this regard focuses particularly upon how women use their sexual capacity. Nevertheless, despite the greater severity applied to women, female sexual satisfaction remains valued as a necessary prerequisite to fertility, and fertility is probably the foremost value in Rwandan culture. There is thus a contradictory tendency inherent in the culture both to encourage, and to fear, healthy female sexuality.

While in the Rwandan capital of Kigali, I listened to a radio program concerning AIDS. The radio commentator, a man, seemed to place the entire responsibility for the spread of the disease upon females. Female prostitution and female conjugal infidelity were the primary reasons for the spread of AIDS, he maintained, and should be strictly discouraged. It did not seem to occur to him that men frequent female prostitutes, nor that more often Rwandan men are unfaithful to their wives than vice versa. My point is not so much that the commentator was wrong in laying the blame for AIDS upon women, as much as that he was relying upon an old cultural attitude concerning the nature of female sexuality to explain a new problem. Despite the newness of the "disease" of AIDS, the "illness" of AIDS has been, in part, culturally prefabricated. Hence, as in the poster described earlier in this chapter, an infected woman is chasing a reluctant man.

## CONCLUSION

Societies around the world with a high HIV seroprevalence have tended to construct illness metaphors about the sickness in very specific ways. These metaphors often strike more at emotionality than at rationality, but they can be understood by looking closely at the society's history and culture. Illness metaphors draw social and moral boundaries between the imagined states of civility and disorder. They describe both the disruptive forces societies fear from outside their borders, as well as the subversive forces societies fear from within. Furthermore, these illness metaphors influence the course of action that social systems take to combat disease, for whether a society responds attentively or with indifference to a disease depends in large part upon its perception of the status of those who suffer from it. In some instances these metaphors become part of the problem, part of the pathogenic process associated with disease. Responsible health policy thus entails curing society of its "illnesses," as well as of its "diseases."

While it seems useful to denounce the process of constructing potentially harmful illness metaphors as Sontag (1977) has done, it is also naive. The process of attributing social and moral values to the largely fortuitous occurrence of contracting disease is probably an inevitable corollary to social existence. Instead, an attempt must be made to understand the specific cultural logic that underlies these metaphors. Even if metaphoric elaboration cannot be avoided with certain sicknesses, we should remember that metaphors can be changed, and that hopefully, we can discourage the tendency to blame our diseases on scapegoats. While no effort should be spared in attempting to understand AIDS as a "disease," we also need to comprehend AIDS as an "illness," and this means attempting to understand society and culture.

## NOTE

1. The term "sickness" will be used throughout this chapter whenever it is unnecessary to rigorously distinguish between "disease" and "illness."

## REFERENCES

Barnouw, E., and Clark, E.G., "Syphilis: The Invader," Public Affairs Pamphlet no. 24, Columbia University Press, New York, 1955.

Berger, P., and Luckman, T., *The Social Construction of Reality*, Anchor Books, New York, 1967.

Coulter, H., *AIDS and Syphilis: the Hidden Link*, Washington, D.C.: North Atlantic Books, 1987.

Douglas, M., *Purity and Danger*, Routledge and Kegan Paul, London, 1966.

Eatough, G., *Fracastoro's Syphilis*. Classical and Medieval Texts, Papers and Monographs 12, Francis Cairns, Liverpool, 1984.

Gaignebet, C., and Florentin, M.C., *Le Carnaval*, Payot, Paris, 1974.

Gould, S.J., *The Mismeausre of Man*, Norton & Co., New York, 1981.

de Heusch, L., *Rois nés d'un coeur de vache*. Gallimard, Paris, 1982.

Kleinman, A., *Patients and Healers in the Context of Culture*. University of California Press, Berkeley, 1980.

Kleinman, A., Eisenberg, L., and Good, B., "Culture, Illness and Care: Clinical Lessons from Anthropologic and Cross-Cultural Research," *Annals of Internal Medicine*, vol. 88, 1978: 251–58.

Lovejoy, A., *The Great Chain of Being*. Harvard University Press, Cambridge, 1936.

Shilts, R., *And the Band Played On*, St. Martin's Press, New York, 1988.

Smith, P., *Le récit populaire au Rwanda*, Armand Colin, Paris, 1975.

———., "L'efficacité des interdits," *L'Homme*, vol. 19, no. 1, janv.-mars, 1979: 5–47.

Sontag, S., *Illness as Metaphor*, Farrar, Straus and Giroux, New York, 1977.

Taylor, C., "Milk, Honey, and Money: Changing Concepts of Pathology in Rwandan Popular Medicine," Ph.D. diss., Univ. of Virginia, Aug. 1988.

Turner, V., *The Ritual Process*, Cornell University Press, Ithaca, 1969.

Wallerstein, I., *The Modern World System*, Academic Press, New York, 1976.

# Chapter Six

## AIDS and Accusation: Haiti, Haitians, and the Geography of Blame

### Paul Farmer

The Republic of Haiti's role in the AIDS epidemic has been unique and unenviable. In *Blaming Others: Prejudice, Race and Worldwide AIDS*, Sabatier (1988:44,48) notes that "two parts of the developing world, Haiti and Africa, have received widespread publicity as the possible birthplace of AIDS. Haiti, a Caribbean nation whose people are racially of African descent, was singled out first." Sabatier begins to document the effects of this quest for origins on a vast continent and on a tiny island nation. "Today," she concludes, "medical opinion has totally abandoned the idea that AIDS originated in Haiti." What transpired between hypothesis and conclusion? What effects did these speculations have on Haitians, in Haiti and abroad? This chapter attempts to answer these questions, and to describe one rural community's initial response to the advent of AIDS. When taken together, the large-scale and the local bring into sharp relief several methodological and ethical dilemmas often evaded in both biomedical and anthropological investigations of AIDS.

## HAITI AND THE POLITICS OF RISK

"In the annals of medicine, this categorization of a nationality as a 'risk group' is unique" (Dr. Robert Auguste, Haitian Coalition on AIDS, December 1983). In November 1981, just a few months after what would later be termed AIDS was first reported in the medical literature, a number of Haitian immigrants had been seen in Florida hospitals with infections characteristic of the syndrome. Several more cases were soon reported among Haitians living in the New York area. The U.S. Centers for Disease Control (CDC) announced, in July 1982, that 34 "Haitians residing in the United States" had been stricken with opportunistic infections (CDC 1982). In the same year, Canadian officials also learned of such infections in a Haitian immigrant. In a study published in January 1983, Viera and colleagues described AIDS in 40 "previously well" Haitian-Americans, many of whom were recent immigrants. Pitchenik et al. (1983) reported "a new acquired immunodeficiency state," detailing opportunistic infections in "20 Haitian patients living in the Miami-Dade area in Florida." Ten cases in Haitian-born persons were soon reported from Montreal, Canada (Ernst et al. 1983; LeBlanc et al. 1983).

Unlike other patients meeting diagnostic criteria for AIDS, these Haitian immigrants denied that they had engaged in homosexual activity or intravenous drug use. Most had never had a blood transfusion. Almost all other cases of the syndrome known at the time implicated one or more of these "risk factors." The CDC therefore inferred that Haitians per se were in some way at risk for AIDS. Within weeks, the popular press seized this inference as a news item. The press drew upon readily available images of squalor, voodoo, and boatloads of "economic refugees," and thus the addition of "Haitians" to the risk groups opened the way to innumerable unflattering portrayals of both Haitians and Haitian-Americans. In a review of the response of the U.S. press to the AIDS epidemic, Albert (1986:174–75) skeptically notes that Haitian-Americans "present pre-existing characteristics of an already non-normative character. They are black, tend to be poor, are recent immigrants, and the association of Haiti with cult-religious practices fuels the current tendency to see deviance in groups at-risk for AIDS." Somehow, it all fit so nicely.

But there was more. In a calculus of blame that uncannily recalled the diplomatic quarantine that greeted the founding in 1804 of the world's first black republic, the disease was presumed to have *come from* Haiti. Gilman suggests that the associative logic ran like this:

The fact that AIDS was found among heterosexuals in Haiti could only be evidence that Haiti was the *source* of the disease. Heterosexual transmission was labeled by investigators as a more "primitive" or "atavistic" stage of the development of AIDS. The pattern of infection in the US, where the disease existed only among marginal groups (including blacks), was understood as characterizing a later phase of the disease's history. (Gilman 1988:102)

The effects of these speculations upon Haiti were disastrous. "Nowhere in the hemisphere is poverty so harsh," blared *US News and World Report* on October 31, 1983. "Now the backlash of the AIDS scare is making it worse." But the anti-Haitian backlash may have been felt as keenly in places like New York. Tales of harassment ricocheted through the city's large disaspora community: one heard of mothers who would not let their children attend schools with Haitian-American students, of Haitian cab drivers who had learned to maintain they were from Martinique or Guadeloupe, of families evicted from rented housing for having "black skin and French names," of abrupt firings and interminable quests for jobs for which Haitian-born applicants were "just not right."

A New York schoolteacher related that "children of Haitian origin are being taunted in the school because of the connection in the scientific literature and the public media between Haitians and AIDS" (quoted in Sencer 1983:25). A physician working at a Brooklyn hospital reported that "on several occasions we have received phone calls from prospective employers of Haitians asking if it was safe to employ them" (Landesman 1983:35). Gilman (1988:102) might not be exaggerating when he suggests that "to be Haitian and living in New York City meant that you were perceived as an AIDS 'carrier.' "

Haitians living in the United States and Canada were quick to sense the prejudices that underpinned many of these responses:

The AIDS epidemic came at a time when the U.S. government policy, as evidenced by Coast Guard interdiction of Haitian vessels and by the prolonged incarceration of new Haitian arrivals in Krome and other camps, seemed to most Haitians to single them out as special targets of a racist and exclusionary attitude pervasive in this country. (Nachman and Dreyfuss 1986:33)

By 1984, it has become clear to the newly formed AIDS Discrimination Unit of the New York City Commission on Human Rights that the effects of the risk-group classification on the local Haitian community were "devastating." One member of the unit reported that "Haitian children have been beaten up (and in at least one case, shot) in school; Haitian store owners have gone bankrupt as their businesses failed; and Haitian families have been evicted from their homes" (quoted in Sabatier 1988:47).

Similar stories appeared concerning their tribulations in Canada and elsewhere in the United States. A social service organization in South Florida reported that, following the inclusion of Haitians on the CDC listing, it was suddenly unable to find job placements for a majority of its clients.[1] The organization also received hate mail, which conveyed such slogans as "Hire a Haitian—Help Spread AIDS," and "There was no AIDS in the USA until the illegal criminal Haitian dogs came." Several of these were signed "United Taxpayers Association." Casper (1986:201) cites a poignant example of the effects of the AIDS stigma on Haitian-Americans: "A Haitian man without AIDS states: 'People avoid shaking my hand when they know I'm Haitian. And my wife and I won't speak Haitian at the laundromat because other people are afraid to use the same machine as us. We can pass as Jamaican.' " Syndicated columnist Ann Landers leapt to the defense of a light-skinned Haitian woman whose South American husband had taken, in recent months, to introducing her as French. As Dr. Jeffrey Viera, the senior author of the 1983 paper that helped to put Haitians on the risk list, later remarked,

The original reports of AIDS among Haitian immigrants were sensationalized and misrepresented in the popular press. Some news broadcasts pictured scantily clad black natives dancing frenetically about ritual fires, while others caricatured Haitians with AIDS as illegal aliens and interned in detention camps. The fact that the majority of the Haitian AIDS victims fit neither of these stereotypes was ignored. The impression left with the public in many instances was that AIDS was pervasive throughout the Haitian community. Unlike the homosexual or drug addict, the Haitian was a highly visible victim of the epidemic who could be singled out by virtue of his ethnic and cultural features. (Viera 1985:97)

Dr. Viera was joined by many other researchers in pinning the blame on the media. But the popular press was in many ways upstaged by the scientific community. On December 1, 1982, Dr. Bruce Chabner of the National Cancer Institute made the following statement, which was widely reported: "Homosexuals in New York take vacations in Haiti, and we suspect that this may be an epidemic Haitian virus that was brought back to the homosexual population in the United States."[2] In a letter published in the February 28, 1983 edition of *New York Daily News*, Viera admits that, in the course of an interview he gave to a wire service, "references to voodoo were made in the context of a discussion of theoretical means of transmission of putative infectious agent among susceptible individuals." It was speculated that the disease might be transmitted by voodoo rites, the ingestion of sacrificial animal blood, the eating of cats, ritualized homosexuality, and so on—a rich panoply of exotica. In March 1983, the United States Public Health Service even recommended that Haitian-Americans not donate blood.

Much "medical" writing on AIDS conflates the issues of prevalence and origins. For example, Siegal and Siegal (1983:85) offer what they call "compelling" evidence of the link between Haiti and the origin of the U.S. AIDS epidemic: three cases of transfusion-related transmission (only one of which, date unspecified, took place in Haiti), and the case of a former nun whose sole sexual contact was said to have been in Haiti, where she worked for 30 years. She died in Canada in 1981 "of a disease that her doctors retrospectively recognized as AIDS." According to the authors, these "compelling" data "suggest that the disease is quite prevalent in Haiti; that it predated AIDS in the United States; and that it may be endemic there" (Siegal and Siegal 1983:85). Moore and LeBaron (1986:81, 84) published a speculative paper attempting to construct an argument that AIDS originated in Haiti. Also, the official organ of the American Medical Association saw fit to publish a consideration of these theories under the melodramatic title "Night of the Living Dead" (Greenfield 1986).[3]

Gay men, users of intravenously administered narcotics, those afflicted with an inherited blood-clotting disorder, and an entire nation, largely black: this was the "Four-H Club" of the press and popular humor. The stigma thereby cast on these groups, three of which were already beleaguered by prejudice, has yet to be gauged. But the Haitians were branded not because of bad luck, but because of bad science. Culturally obtuse questionnaires and interviews had yielded, not surprisingly, a long list of "patient denies" for behaviors known to place individuals at risk for AIDS. It was not until later that this research was seriously challenged within the scientific community—and then only at the insistence of the stigmatized. Physicians and leaders of the Haitian-American communities in New York and South Florida formed coalitions in order to counter what they took to be a racist and specifically anti-Haitian stance. "The response of public health officials and AIDS researchers to Haitian protest has ranged," noted Nachman and Dreyfuss (1986:33), "from outrage to sympathetic understanding." Under considerable pressure from Haitian-American community leaders, the New York City Department of Health excised "Haitian" from its official list of "risk groups" in the summer of 1983. The CDC resisted, but in April 1985 it too at last removed, without comment, the term "Haitian" as a risk-group designation.[4] The category has yet to be removed from the list now firmly established in the popular imagination. As one Haitian-American physician complained, "after all the wild theories of voodoo rites and genetic predisposition were aired and dispelled, and the slipshod scientific investigations were brought to light, the public perception of the problem has remained the same—that if Haitians have AIDS, it is very simply because they are Haitians" (quoted in Smith 1983:46).

But regardless of the publicity about Haitians in the U.S. press, AIDS had indeed come to Haiti. Cases of Kaposi's sarcoma, dating as early as June 1979, had been reported in an international medical conference held in Haiti in April 1982 (Liautaud et al. 1982). Several cases of inexplicable opportunistic infection were also presented. These suggestions of immunosuppression were of course strikingly similar to those termed "AIDS" in the North American medical literature, and led to the formation, in May 1982, of the Haitian Study Group on Kaposi's Sarcoma and Opportunistic Infections. A year later, at the Haitian Medical Association's annual meeting in Port-au-Prince, AIDS was the featured topic. The politics of the syndrome, rather than its etiology, prognosis, or clinical management, seemed to dominate the discussions. Reliable clinical research left little doubt that the "infectious agent" was established in and around the capital. A number of researchers from the United States attended, including Dr. Jeffrey Viera; his public apology, though doubtless appreciated, did nothing to counter the collapse of Haiti's important tourist industry, already a fait accompli.

Throughout the 1970s, as international memories of Papa Doc Duvalier began to fade, tourism began to assume increasing importance in Haiti's economy. By 1980, it had become the country's second largest source of foreign currency, and generated employment for thousands living in and around Port-au-Prince. The effects of the "AIDS scare" were dramatic and prompt: the Haitian Bureau of Tourism estimated a decline from 75,000 visitors in the winter of 1982–83 to under 10,000 the following year. Six hotels folded, and as many more were on the edge of bankruptcy. In a letter to the medical journal that had published several of the papers linking AIDS to his country, the Haitian ambassador to the United States declared that "the negative impact on our already distraught economy has been tremendous." Outside assessments concurred: "Already suffering from an image problem, Haiti has been made an international pariah by AIDS," concluded one 1983 report. "Boycotted by tourists and investors, it has lost millions of dollars and hundreds of jobs at a time when half the work force is jobless. Even exports are being shunned by some" (Chaze 1983).

Of course fluctuations in tourism and trade may be attributed to many factors, but there was little doubt in Haiti as to what the cause of the collapse had been: Haiti had been accused of "starting the AIDS epidemic." At the Port-au-Prince medical conference, however, the accusations ran the other way. Haitian and Haitian-American researchers suggested that a significant percentage of those tourists had been gay men from North America. They had come to Haiti to find inexpensive sex, and had brought a North American disease with them.[5] That was why the majority of Haiti's AIDS cases came from the suburb of Carrefour, an important locus of both male and female prostitution. One Haitian-American researcher read aloud from the pages of the 1983 *Spartacus International Gay Guide*, in which Haiti was enthusiastically recommended to the gay tourist: handsome men with "a great ability to satisfy" are readily available, but "there is no free sex in Haiti, except with other gay tourists you may come across. Your partners will expect to be paid for their services but the charges are nominal." Another advertisement, which ran in *The Advocate* ("The National Gay News Magazine"), assured the prospective tourist that Haiti is "a place where all your fantasies come true" (Moore and LeBaron 1986:82).

But if AIDS in Haiti was transmitted through homosexual contact, why were the sex differences in the epidemiology of the syndrome less striking in Haiti than in the United States and Europe? Although 88 percent of the initial Haitian cases were among men, more and more women were diagnosed with AIDS each year. By 1983, women accounted for between a quarter and a third of all cases reported by Haitian investigators. Haitian researchers suggested that Haitian male prostitutes did not consider themselves homosexual, but were desperate for money. They were often married, or involved in relationships with women. Thus AIDS was introduced to Haiti by contact between North American gay men and *bisexual* Haitian men. This was held to explain, in part, the rapidly declining percentage of men with AIDS in Haiti, as well as the decreasing importance of homosexual transmission.[6] Furthermore, the rate of transfusion-associated transmission was much higher in Haiti than in the United States, and Haitian women are more likely to receive blood—often in the course of an obstetrical intervention—than are Haitian men. Fully 40 percent of Haitian women diagnosed with AIDS between 1982 and 1984 had received at least one unit of blood, usually from paid donors (Pape 1985, 1987; Pape et al. 1986).

The Haitian Medical Association came down hard on the CDC, deploring its "unscientific and racist attitude [which] only reflects the inability of the CDC to define high-risk groups in the Haitian population."[7] Dr. Jean Pape, one of Haiti's leading AIDS researchers, is equally critical:

The categorisation of Haitians, with homosexuals and drug addicts, in a separate 'risk group' was a serious error in the interpretation of the epidemiological data. The CDC never wondered why 88 percent of the early Haitian AIDS cases in the U.S. occurred in males. In 1983 our group had identified risk factors, bisexuality and blood transfusion, in 79 percent of Haitian AIDS patients. (cited in Sabatier 1988:45)

One question left largely untouched and entirely unresolved by the Haitian physicians was an epidemiologic one: If AIDS had its center of transmission in urban areas like Carrefour, had it spread to rural Haiti? One spokesman for the association suggested, in a telephone interview with the *New York Times*, that AIDS did not occur among Haitian peasants.[8] His assertion was not based on epidemiologic research, however, but on the fact that virtually all known cases of AIDS had been among city-dwellers. The same might be said for virtually all AIDS research, which had at that time been conducted exclusively in and around the capital.

Given that a reliable test for the virus, or for antibodies to it, did not exist at the time, diagnosis was made on the basis of clinical signs and symptoms. The most important of these, Haitian researchers reported, were chronic diarrhea, weight loss, and intermittent fever. These are very common symptoms in Haiti, and would not be enough to differentiate AIDS from various gastrointestinal disorders, tuberculosis, tropical spure (a malabsorption disorder), and several other infectious diseases—especially given the synergistic effect of malnutrition, widespread in Haiti. Further, the most common presenting infection in Haitians with AIDS was reported to be tuberculosis, already endemic before the arrival of the virus. And so AIDS in the countryside was a mystery. This was—quite inappropriately—a comfort to those of us working in rural area. Given the case fatality rate, perhaps it is understandable that Haitian clinicians, like the population in general, seemed to need to think of the disease as a "city sickness." Such, in any case, was the attitude in the village I shall call "Do Kay."

## AIDS COMES TO A HAITIAN VILLAGE

*Sida?* Yes, of course I've heard of it. It's caused by living in the city. It gives you diarrhea and can kill you. . . . We've never had *sida* here. It's a city sickness (*maladi lavil*). (Pierre F., 27, schoolteacher, in a July 1985 interview)

It was *sida* that killed him: that's what I'm trying to tell you. But they say it was a death sent to him. They sent a *sida* death to him . . . *sida* is caused by a tiny microbe. But not just anybody will catch the microbe that can cause *sida*. (Pierre F. in a September 1987 interview)

The village of Do Kay stretches along an unpaved road that cuts through Haiti's Central Plateau. Consisting in 1987 of approximately 800 persons, Do Kay is composed primarily of peasant farmers who were displaced some 30 years ago by the construction of Haiti's largest dam. Before 1957, the village of Kay was situated near the banks of a larger river. When the valley was flooded to build a hydroelectric dam, the majority of villagers were forced up into the hills on either side of the new reservoir. Kay became divided into "Do" (those who settled on the stony backs of the hills) and "Ba" (those who remained down near the new waterline). By all the standard measures, both parts of Kay are now very poor; its older inhabitants often blame their poverty on the massive buttress dam a few miles away, and note that it brought them neither electricity nor water. The sole improvements in their lives, they observe, have been the construction of a school and a clinic built and run by Père Jacques Alexis,[9] a Haitian Episcopal priest who has been working in the area for over 30 years.

When I first began working in Do Kay, in May 1983, the word *sida* (from the French acronym S.I.D.A.) was just beginning to work its way into the rural Haitian lexicon. For example, in interviews I conducted in the first months of 1984, only one of 17 informants mentioned *sida* as a possible cause of diarrhea. When questioned, however, 15 of the 17 had heard of *sida*; 12 of them offered characteristics of the disorder. Although there was some disagreement as to what those characteristics might be, the following assessment, from a 36-year-old market woman, was not atypical of descriptions elicited in 1984: "*Sida* is a sickness they have in Port-au-Prince and in the United States. It gives you a diarrhea that starts very slowly, but never stops until you're completely dry. There's no water left in your body. . . . *Sida* is a sickness that you see in men who sleep with other men."

Although two persons suggested that "*sida* is the same thing as tuberculosis," most of those questioned mentioned three attributes: the novelty of *sida*, its relation to diarrhea, and its association with homosexuality. The villagers who offered such a description had heard of AIDS on the radio or during trips to the capital. Less than three years later, ideas about the disorder and its origin had changed drastically. The case of Manno Surpris in particular seems to have influenced their views. Manno moved to Do Kay in 1982, when he became a teacher at Père Jacques's large new school. He was 25 years old.

Born in a small village in another part of the Central Plateau, Manno was the son of peasant farmers. After having passed his primary school exams, he moved to Mirebalais, a large market town not far from his home village, and there he began his secondary school education. Several months after his arrival, he left to complete his secondary education in the capital. As is often the case for rural children with such expectations, Manno did odd jobs in order to pay tuition at one of what many urban Haitians label "lottery schools" (so-called because, as far as learning is concerned, "you take your chances there.") In five years, Manno completed only two more grades. Concluding that he would never be able to complete his studies, Manno moved back to Mirebalais, hoping to find a job.

Well before Père Jacques Alexis completed the school he was building at Do Kay, he began looking for teachers interested in working with villagers. He knew that *lycee* graduates would not be easy to recruit, so he was happy to offer a position to Manno, who had the equivalent of an eighth-grade education.

Less than a year after his arrival, Manno had become Père Jacques's favorite teacher, and within two years had been entrusted by the priest with a number of public responsibilities. Manno was put in charge of the new village pig pen, and was made responsible for the maintenance of the water pump on which the community depended for all of its water. As Père Jacques later recalled, "I felt that he was good-natured and dependable. But most of all, he didn't seem to be in as much of a hurry to get back to Mirebalais on Friday afternoon. He really seemed to like working in the village." Alourdes Monestime, also a teacher, was one reason that Manno enjoyed staying at Do Kay. In 1984 their daughter was born; a year later, they began building their own house not far from the school. A second child was on the way.

I knew that Manno was not universally popular. He was a salaried teacher; some of his other duties were also remunerative, and so he was confronted by the envy of the less fortunate. This jealousy was compounded by the fact that for the villagers he was *moun vini*, a "newcomer" or "outsider." That at least one person resented Manno's status was made obvious when, shortly after Baby Doc Duvalier's departure in February 1986, Manno's half-finished house was knocked down. Although these kinds of events were common throughout Haiti, this was the only such incident in the Kay area. The significance of the sentiment against him was not clear to me until August, when Manno beat an adolescent schoolboy for some transgression in the pigsty.

I was quite surprised by the intensity of the community's reaction to the beating. The "facts" were quickly circulated by word of mouth: the schoolboy had inadvertently let several pigs escape. Upon discovering this, Manno attacked him with a length of rubber hose. The elderly man who had unofficially adopted the boy upon the death of his mother was not in the village, and a couple of local men were muttering about settling the score with Manno themselves. Someone sent word to the boy's grandmother, who lived a couple of hours from Do Kay. A couple of schoolboys began carrying their own lengths of hose "for self-defense." The crisis was defused by Mme. Alexis, Père Jacques' wife; she called for a meeting between the adults concerned (Manno, the child's grandmother, and the foster parent at Do Kay). During this meeting, Manno apologized to the boy. With the apology, I thought that the whole affair was closed.

After a day or two, I heard no more grumbling against Manno. Perhaps the grumbling had ended because he had fallen ill. Before the incident, Manno had been bothered by intermittent diarrhea. He had been plagued with superficial skin infections throughout the summer. The patches would clear up with treatment, only to appear again, usually on the scalp, neck, or face. Early in the fall, Père Jacques took Manno twice to see a dermatologist in Port-au-Prince. Manno's diarrhea had come and gone and come again. His weight loss had become evident even to casual acquaintances. By December, his decline was drastic, and Manno began to cough. Père Jacques took him to Port-au-Prince again shortly before Christmas. Manno saw one of the country's best-known internists, who ordered a chest x-ray and tuberculosis skin test.

By Christmas, the staff of the Do Kay clinic began to whisper, among themselves, that AIDS could be the cause of Manno's problems, but said nothing to Père Jacques. Manno was seeing an eminent physician, they reasoned; he would certainly not overlook such an obvious possibility. After the New Year, each day brought a noticeable decline in Manno's health. At the same time a rumor was circulating around Do Kay: Manno was the victim of some sort of evil. His illness was the intentional result of some angry or jealous rival. I heard this rumor from an 18-year-old former student of Manno's. He would not tell me who had passed on this gossip to him, and attempted to dismiss it: "I don't believe it myself; but that's what some people say." He also said he did not know who would wish to harm Manno. I asked by what means he thought such an illness could have been inflicted on Manno, and again the student was vague. "I don't know . . . some people can do it by themselves, some go to a *bokor*" [a voodoo practitioner adept with powers to heal and to harm].

Having been exposed in the ethnographic literature to dramatic descriptions of "voodoo death" in Haiti and elsewhere, I worried about the effects of this rumor on Manno's health. Had he heard it as well? When I broached the subject with Mme. Alexis, I found that she also knew of it, and she had heard the story from Alourdes herself. "But once a real diagnosis is given, every one will understand that this is not a case of evil done to him." She stated this in mid-January, while Manno was being evaluated by the distinguished internist. Everyone agreed that a diagnosis was needed. Although Manno appeared to be dying, all of the doctor's expensive tests had been negative. Upon inquiry, I discovered that Père Jacques had, by this time, already considered the possibility of AIDS. Madame Alexis, who had not, was shocked at the suggestion. "But how on earth could he have contracted that illness? . . . He's been married for three years," she protested. "And surely, he isn't homosexual?"

After two months of wavering; the internist referred Manno to the country's sole public AIDS clinic. By the time Manno went there, the clinic had closed for the weekend. But would Manno last until Monday? He could no longer walk, was dehydrated, weighed less than 90 pounds, and was disoriented. Père Jacques suggested that he spend the weekend in Mirebalais rather than Do Kay. He could be made more comfortable, it was thought, in one of the houses that were then being used as dormitories for villagers who were studying at the town *lycee*.

Manno did survive the weekend. On Monday I was asked to take him to Port-au-Prince. We reached the clinic by midmorning; it was already crowded with emaciated men and women. Because Manno was among the most sickly looking, we were seen almost immediately. A young AIDS specialist looked at Manno, and then at the x-ray we had brought with us from the previous workup. She questioned him in Creole and then turned to me and said in perfect English: "I don't understand [the referring doctor's] verdict. I read this as a clear-cut case of disseminated tuberculosis." She paused and then added, "I'm afraid the [HIV-antibody] test will prove positive; regardless, you've got a very sick man on your hands. We'll draw the blood for the [HIV-antibody] test, and start him on [antituberculous medications]."

We returned to Mirebalais with all prescriptions filled. Within three days Manno no longer looked like a dying man. He spoke easily and seemed grateful for the visits that only a few days before had seemed only to confuse him. His cough persisted, but was less incessant, and he began eating. As he began to improve, I was finally able to spend time alone with him. In an interview conducted in the first week of February, before we received the results of the HIV-antibody test, I asked him what he thought had made him so sick. Manno looked embarrassed and troubled. "Well, I don't really know . . . I don't know." "What are you most afraid of?" Tears came to his eyes. He knows, I thought. He knows that he might have AIDS. Instead, he replied: "Most of all, I hope it's not tuberculosis. But I'm afraid that's what it is. I'm coughing, I've lost weight . . . I'm afraid I have tuberculosis, and that I'll never get better, never be able to work again. . . . People don't want to be near you if you have tuberculosis."

It was during this time, too, that Manno shared with me the history of his sexual activity. For a 30-year old man who was thought to have AIDS, his reported sexual activity was strikingly sparse, especially when compared to those elicited from North Americans with AIDS, or to their HIV-seronegative, age-matched controls.[10] Manno reported sexual contact with only four persons, all of them women. None of them was involved in prostitution. Two of these women he met in Port-au-Prince, the third in Mirebalais, and the fourth was Alourdes, whom he had met at Do Kay in 1982. Since he became involved with Alourdes about four years ago, he said, he had slept with no one else. He reported never having had sexual contact with a man or boy; he denied use of any narcotics (indeed, he had heard of neither heroin nor marijuana, although he was familiar with the Haitian word for "illicit drug."). He had received, However, "at least a dozen" intramuscular injections, usually of penicillin or injectable vitamins. Although many of these had been administered in the preceding months, several injections were given years ago. He had never received a transfusion; the intravenous fluids he had received in the past month had been administered with sterile needles.

According to the national laboratory, Manno did indeed have HIV antibodies. He also had tuberculosis, and responded very well to the antituberculous regimen. On his next trip to see the doctor, Alourdes went with him. She tested seronegative, and the doctor advised her to avoid unprotected sexual contact with Manno. The doctor informed both of them that Manno had AIDS, but that she would do everything in her power to help him fight off the infections commonly seen in Haitians with AIDS.

Manno remained in Mirebalais for over a month. Although disheartened by the lab results and fully aware of the usual course of the disease, Père Jacques spared no expense in treating Manno: prescriptions were filled promptly, well-balanced meals were prepared and delivered, the staff of the clinic at Do Kay were encouraged to visit Manno regularly. His mother came from their home village; Alourdes's sister came from a village near Do Kay. Everyone took turns taking care of Manno. No one seemed afraid to touch him, although family members had been warned that Manno's illness was "caused by a microbe." By late February Manno was going for walks, and he had put on 20 pounds. He had stopped coughing completely. By mid-March, he no longer looked ill at all. Père Jacques wondered whether or not Manno might return to teaching by the fall semester. Mme. Alexis was sure that he had been misdiagnosed, despite warnings from the staff doctor that his apparent recovery was in keeping with the course of the disease.

Manno did so well, in fact, that his neighbors and coworkers soon began to wonder why he had not returned to Do Kay. If no one seemed particularly leery of Manno, the same could not be said of Manno himself. He was frightened of something, or someone. His wife returned to the area before him. But when Alourdes returned to her teaching post, she chose to stay at her mother's house— almost an hour's dusty walk from the school. When I asked Père Jacques why Manno was reluctant to return to Kay, he responded candidly:

I have heard that Manno believes that he is the victim of someone's ill-will. I hope you can at least see why this sort of accusation is dangerous. It doesn't hurt anyone if you blame a microbe, but blaming someone else for your misfortunes leads to division and hatred. That's why I'm so unhappy that Manno believes he's been the victim of evil.

Père Jacques's "unhappiness" may have resulted in a confrontation between him and Manno. In any case, the latter's departure from Mirebalais was surreptitious. Père and Mme. Alexis later expressed their disapprobation of Manno's "lack of personality." He should at least have come by before leaving Mirebalais," Père Jacques complained, "but I haven't seen him at all."

Manno was indeed difficult to track down. In March, I traveled to Alourdes's mother's house at least three times; her son-in-law was never there. He was "in his own country, at his mother's," or he was "in Mirebalais for a couple of days." These responses seemed fine to me, and I would have kept on believing them, if one of my coworkers had not lived next door to Alourdes's mother. Community health worker Christian Guerrier was also related to Alourdes: his father and her father were brothers. The day after my third futile visit; Christian explained to me that there was much that I did not understand:

There's something you need to understand about Haitians, at least some of them. They believe that there are different kinds of medications for different kinds of illnesses. Some illnesses require several different kinds of medication. . . . Manno is not at his mother's house. He is in Vieux Fonds [a small village, about two hours' walk from Do Kay] being treated by a voodoo priest (houngan). He believes that, because someone sent him the illness, it must be taken away.

Christian observed that Manno's treatment might take a long time—"many days or weeks." I would not see him until the houngan had finished treating him.

Finally, Christian intimated that I might wish to confront Alourdes about her husband's whereabouts, taking care not to let her know that her cousin had revealed the true nature of Manno's absence.

In a subsequent interview, Alourdes did not seem reluctant to impart more detailed information about Manno's treatment. At first, she was careful to attribute his activities to "his own beliefs" about his illness: "Manno believes that they did this to him because they were jealous that he had three jobs—teaching, the pigsty, and the water pump." Later in the same interview, however, she dropped all pretense at skepticism: "The people who did this to him already know what they've done; they know what kind of illness they've sent. He won't survive: there are people who know how to send a TB death (*voye yon mo tebe*) on someone; that person gets TB." Alourdes was reluctant to tell me who was responsible for sending the disease, but at last told me,

Yes, you know the people who did this. One comes from my husband's hometown; another comes from here; the third is even related to me, although he pretends that he is not. Two of them work inside the school complex. The one who comes from my husband's country is at the head of it . . . he's the master of the affair, he arranged it.

I knew that one of the schoolteachers, Fritz, was from the same town as Manno and asked if it was he who bewitched him. Alourdes nodded, and then she quickly added that another teacher was the second member of the group. She adamantly refused to name the third. I discovered only later that the triad was completed by her cousin, Christian's sister—and Fritz's fiancée.

Knowledge of the family's suspicion of sorcery seemed to be widespread. Mme. Alexis brought up the subject on several occasions and continued to express her exasperation over "their persistent superstition": "I know people believe that someone can send someone a tuberculous death, but how can they think such a thing when they know the diagnosis? I was sure that when the family received the [HIV-antibody] test results they would abandon the notion that a person was responsible."

A full month elapsed before I saw Manno again. In early May, I stopped by his wife's mother's house. The family owned two small houses, built side by side with a granary between them. One of them had been emptied for Manno and his family. When I reached the yard, I saw that Manno was lying inside the house in bed, but he jumped to his feet when I greeted him, "Manno, I never seem to see you." His handshake was firm; he had put on at least another 15 pounds. "Oh, you know, I just don't seem to get down to Do Kay." If Manno's medical condition had temporarily improved, his social dilemma had not. He and his family blamed close friends for what they feared to be an inevitably fatal illness. He had abandoned his house, and estranged Père Jacques, his and his wife's employer. By late June, when he began to develop diarrhea and fever, I learned from Christian that Manno and his family were increasingly obsessed, not with the course of the disease, but with its ultimate origin. Until he was willing to speak more candidly with me about his suspicions, the course of the disease remained the chief focus of our discussions.

The subject was finally broached on a day during which Manno had an appointment with his physician in Port-au-Prince. I found Manno waiting for a bus. I offered to give him a ride to Mirebalais, where he could more easily catch a bus for Port-au-Prince. While on the road back to Do Kay and Mirebalais, I asked, "Tell me more about your illness—the sort of things we haven't been able to talk about for lack of privacy." His response was equally direct: "I know that I am very sick, even though I don't look it. They tell me there's no cure. But I'm not sure of that. If you can find a cause, you can find a cure." When I asked, "What is the cause of your illness?" Manno unhesitatingly replied, "A microbe" (*mikwòb*). Because silence followed this response, I asked him, "Why aren't you staying in your house?" "Well, my mother-in-law suggested that we move in with her until I was feeling better." "But you've been feeling better for months now," I answered. "Yes," he said after a pause. "That's true."

We had been through this already, more than once, and I decided to press him. "It has been suggested," I remarked, "that you moved out of your house because you thought someone from Do Kay was trying to harm you." Manno weighed my question. I began to wonder if he were short of breath, but he answered in a steady voice: 'Perhaps that's what they say, but that doesn't mean it's true. . . . Well, I don't know if someone is trying to harm me, but I don't know that someone isn't. Maybe, maybe not." Manno was clearly not about to divulge more, but we agreed to continue the "frank discussion" the following week.

The summer of 1987 was a difficult period in which to keep appointments. On several occasions, political unrest paralyzed the major cities. Our meeting was cancelled by a strike that shut down most roads. Manno missed at least two more appointments at the AIDS clinic, one because gunfire in the streets scared away the staff and patients. By late July, Manno began complaining again of diarrhea. And his neighbor, Christian, informed me that Manno was coughing again. "Due to the political problems," Manno was unable to refill his supply of one of his antituberculous drugs. By early August, he was vomiting, and complained of "terrible headaches." By the third week in August, Manno was once more gravely ill. A group of young men from Do Kay, most of them my coworkers, asked me to drive them to Manno's house "for a prayer meeting." "We have heard," one of them added, "that he and his wife are in spiritual danger." We reached the house by 9 P.M. and found the family in bed. The children were asleep on their little mat on the floor, and their mother appeared to be sleeping there with them. Manno was in his bed, and he seemed somewhat embarrassed by our visit. When I asked him about his headaches, he described them as "no better, no worse." One visitor initiated a couple of songs; a few fragments of Bible verse were recited. Another person prayed, asking the Almighty to send down his "spiritual medication."

By the end of the month, Manno's breathing had become labored. The painkillers no longer helped and he had not been sleeping. He vomited after most meals and had lost a great deal of weight. In mid-September, Christian informed me that Manno was worse than ever. We reached Manno later in the afternoon. His mother was there, which I took to be a bad sign. Also present were his brother and a cousin, neither of whom I had met before. When I arrived in the yard, I could hear Manno's short, labored breathing. Christian and the others remained outside during the half-hour I was in the house. Manno had great difficulty speaking, but seemed to be lucid. His eyes rolled a bit when he spoke, and he was as thin as he had been in January. I realized that Manno was dying, and my subsequent request seemed hollow. "Let us take Manno to the hospital," I said to his wife's father. "No, no—I'm in the middle of treating him with herbs," he answered evenly but forcefully. "I'll give him to you, but after twenty-one or so days."

Manno died the next morning. I heard the news just before midday, and went immediately to the house. A dozen or so friends and family were sitting quietly under the granary. Alourdes's mother was wailing in the doorway of her house. I found Alourdes inside her mother's front room, sitting on the bed. She looked more tired than grief-stricken. Her little boy was nursing. Manno had not slept last night, said Alourdes, nor had she. He had asked for some cola and milk early in the morning, but vomited it almost immediately. At about 10:30 or so, Manno had complained that he was almost out of breath. This must be due, he felt, to his short rations. So he asked his wife to prepare him a plantain. He was groaning. "A few minutes later, when I noticed he wasn't groaning, I went back in. He had died while I was cooking the plantain."

I sat in the room for a while, on the floor. Someone brought us chairs, and we continued to sit in silence. Finally I decided to leave in order to bring news of the death to Père Jacques, who was visiting a mission station on the far side of the reservoir. I went back over to the other house and asked Alourdes what was going to happen. She replied that the funeral would be the following day. She had commissioned a coffin to be made, and her father had gone off to make arrangements for the grave.

That evening, I went to the wake, There was a good deal of crying and little attempt at the sort of humor I had seen at the wakes of older rural Haitians. Alourdes wrote a note to Père Jacques concerning the funeral. When I returned to Do Kay, however, I found the priest had departed for Mirebalais. The sacraments were left to Gerard, the lay leader of the Do Kay mission and the principal of the school that had employed Manno. By the time Gerard and I returned the next morning, Manno had already been buried. There were no more than a dozen people milling about the yard. Gerard announced that he would offer his "ministrations at the time of death," which meant, I soon discovered, that he would read from a Creole version of The Book of Common Prayer, and hold forth on any lessons to be learned from the brief life of Manno Surpris. When Gerard stepped into the room in which Manno had died, he was followed only by Alourdes, carrying her son, and Manno's mother.

I was very uncomfortable when Gerard called me into the house, where he was lecturing to his polite but distracted audience.

Man cannot hurt man. Manno never hurt anyone; on the contrary, one thing he was known for was his ready smile. So why would someone wish to harm him? It is a very bad thing to accuse someone else of trying to harm him, a very heavy load. No, we all know what illness he had. He had *sida*.

He turned to me and added, "Didn't he?" It was the first time I had heard them publicly confronted with the word *sida*, though there was no one in the family who did not know of the diagnosis. It was not naming the illness that disturbed me, but the fear that Alourdes would think I had betrayed her confidence by discussing the subject with Gerard. At about this time, Alourdes's father entered the room. Gerard might as well have spoken to a mahogany tree, for the man began whispering, in an unabashed way, about the latest signs of malevolence from Fritz. It was never clear that Gerard understood that the family might agree that Manno had died of *sida* but that someone—and the name "Fritz" kept surfacing—had sent the illness "on him."

It seems that wherever AIDS strikes, accusation is never far behind. In the United States, blame and counter-blame played large roles in public discourse on AIDS risk-groups. In at least one Haitian village, however, the calculus of blame was strikingly different from that seen in North America. Noticeably absent was the revulsion with which AIDS patients were faced in North America, in both clinical settings and in their communities. In the United States we read of employers summarily firing persons with AIDS; in rural Haiti we encounter an employer angry because his employee with AIDS is avoiding him. North Americans with AIDS have left eloquent testimony to the meaning of the syndrome there: "You get fired, you get evicted from your apartment. You're a leper. You die alone" (Whitmore 1988:26). This summary is far from describing the experience of Manno, nor would it describe that of the young woman from Do Kay who died of AIDS several months after Manno's death (see Farmer and Kleinman 1989).

This striking difference cannot be ascribed to Haitian "ignorance of modes of transmission." On the contrary, the Haitians I interviewed have ideas of etiology and epidemiology that reflect the incursion of the "North American ideology" of AIDS—that the disease is caused by a virus and is somehow related to homosexuality. There were later subsumed, however, in uniquely Haitian beliefs about illness causation. Long before the advent of AIDS to Do Kay, I should have asked if *sida* could be caused by malevolent magic. Sorcery accusations did not surprise Père and Mme. Alexis, although the latter expressed dismay that such a "false idea" could be held concurrently with "the real cause." Although Père Jacques cast his analysis in terms of the familiar dichotomy of voodoo versus Christianity, my coworkers—who are from Do Kay or surrounding villages—spoke in less dualistic terms. A series of oppositions, rather than one, seemed to guide much of their conversation with me: An illness might be caused by a "microbe" or by magic or by both. Some even spoke of the night, years ago, when Manno had been knocked out of bed by a bolt of lightning. The shock, they said, had left him "susceptible" to a disease caused by a "microbe" and "sent by someone." An illness might be treated by doctors or voodoo priests or herbalists or prayer or any combination of these. The extent to which Manno believed in each of these treatment modalities remains unclear. I believe he was glad to receive all of them.

In considering together the international drama of the epidemic, as told in part in the first section of this chapter, and the drama that unfolded in one small village, one is first struck by the differences between the two tales. But there also emerges a striking similarity between these responses to the advent of AIDS. The quest for *origins* is of great importance in both settings. In both settings, too, the opposition of insider/outsider delineates the contours of a geography of blame. The story of Manno's final year, when read with the help of his moral map, leads us to a number of methodological and ethical questions about the role of anthropology in AIDS research.

## "DO YOU BELIEVE IN VOODOO?": POWER AND ETHICS IN AIDS RESEARCH

It would be ingenuous of the researcher to assume that acquiescence to the request for an interview means that a villager will tell the truth once the interview has started, or that the villager's affability is an indicator of the veracity of what he says. On the contrary, the villager has very good reasons not to tell the truth. Secrecy is one the few effective survival tactics the Haitian peasantry can use against the outside world. There are strong personal norms against revealing one's personal affairs and resources to strangers. (Chen and Murray 1976: 243)

In April 1983, while visiting colleagues in Miami, I was invited by them to examine a proposal for AIDS research that was then being considered for federal funding. This was not a formal request for a review, but an unofficial peek offered by fellow anthropologists exasperated by the crudity of what the authors of the proposal immodestly called 'the research instrument." Thus one question read: Do you consider yourself (check one) _____ heterosexual _____ homosexual. The interview schedule was "to be translated into French." When an anthropologist told the investigators that most Haitians do not speak French, they conceded that, given this fact, Creole should be the language in which interviews would be conducted. Those administering the questionnaire would be asking for histories of a number of sexually transmitted diseases that Haitian entrants knew to be reasons for exclusion from the United States. And where were these data to be sent? To a U.S. government agency! Here are some other queries from a version of the interview schedule:

Which of the following illnesses have you had? (check one)

Kaposi's sarcoma Yes _____ No _____

Pneumocystis pneumonia Yes _____ No _____

CNS toxoplasmosis Yes _____ No _____

Cryptococcal meningitis Yes _____ No _____

Have you ever touched, drunk, or eaten raw milk, blood products, or meat of animals during voodoo rituals or hunting experiences? (check one)

Yes _____ No _____ Unknown _____

How old were you when you first had sexual intercourse with a male (man or boy)? _____ years or never _____ (check here)

Did you ever pay for or were you ever paid by a person to have sex with you? (check one) Yes _____ No _____ Unknown _____

Have you ever had a job or spent some time in a place frequented by homosexual men, e.g., a bathhouse, a gymnasium, gay bar? (check one)

Yes _____ No _____ Unknown _____

It is difficult to think of a challenge more difficult than eliciting from informants the sort of information that is necessary for sound epidemiologic research on AIDS—unless it is the task of eliciting such sensitive information across boundaries of language, culture, and class. I can think of no proposition more immodest than a volley of yes-no questions that would attempt to pierce, in an hour, the complex and private spheres of sexuality, cosmology, the personhood. The fallacy of such methodologies is perhaps most apparent to those who have worked in a society such as Haiti, where there is considerable institutionalized secrecy. The case of Manno Surpris is emblematic, I believe, of the difficulties confronting those who would use questionnaires or closed-ended interviews as the primary means of extracting information. Despite years of friendship between us, it took many hours of open-ended interviewing and just plain visiting, over the course of several months, before several key issues could even be discussed.

The limitations of such methodologies is further illustrated in the manner in which these interview schedules approached the Haitian folk-religious complex. "Do you believe in voodoo?" was a question in the 1983 version of the interview schedule. "Have you ever heard of voodoo?" was a subsequent attempt to make a leading question less obviously so, but it was clear that most AIDS researchers shared the received wisdom: "Although ostensibly Roman Catholic, all Haitians except the educated urban elite (scarcely 10 percent of the population) participate in the voodoo cult, at least by watching the spirit possessions and by dancing in the all night dances that follow the ceremony proper" (Moore and LeBaron 1986:80–81). There seem to be compelling reasons for foreigners, including social scientists and members of the urban Haitian elite, to presume the *universality* of voodoo "beliefs" and "practices" among the peasantry. In fact, we lack any statistically sound assessment of its importance in contemporary Haiti.

With all the good will in the world, such an assessment would be difficult to make, for voodoo also exemplifies the often overlooked link between truth and power. Why might this Haitian religion be shrouded in secrecy? Haitian history is full of periodic "anti-superstition" campaigns against voodoo. And one notes not only home-grown persecution, but those foreign missionaries who are loud and persistent enemies of voodoo. One of them was recently quoted in *Life* magazine as saying, "It is voodoo that is the devil here." He continues, "It is a demonic religion, a cancer on Haiti. Voodoo is worse than AIDS. And it is one of the reasons for the epidemic."[11] When men who make pronouncements such as this one are in positions of power—where access to jobs, food, medical care, and schooling in an impoverished country are to a significant extent in their hands—it becomes easier to see why voodoo surrounds itself with a wall of secrecy (or "lying"). As a number of anthropologists have recently observed, the more the disempowered perceive to be at stake, the greater their incentive to resort to secrecy, especially in the context of religious or cultural persecution (see, for example, Chen and Murray 1976; Nachman 1984:538; Scheper-Hughes 1987:71). And when power is as unevenly distributed as it is in Haiti, a research methodology that ignores the effects of this distribution upon people's willingness to share information might obscure more than it illuminates.

What other reasons for secrecy exist in Haiti? One is made clear in the ethnography presented above: the politics of reputation and envy in small villages. Another reason for secrecy surely stems from the abuses of state power by its local representatives—the *"tonton macoutes"* or the army. In August 1983, the government of Jean-Claude Duvalier began a crackdown on gays in Port-au-Prince. "We have found that most people with AIDS are homosexuals, and that's why we moved against homosexuals," said a government spokesman. The regime proudly announced plans for "a general fight against homosexuality." Another official predicted that "arrested homosexuals can look forward to three to six months in jail and then 'will be sent somewhere to reform them.' No lawyers will defend them, he predicted."[12] Clubs and hotels were also forcibly closed; scores of "homosexuals" were arrested and beaten; a few foreigners were deported.

For many anthropologists working in the Third World, this will have a certain troubling resonance—similar repressive actions have already been taken in several countries. But it is also relevant in the United States, where groups thought to be "at-risk for AIDS" have also been the subjects of persecution. Further, since many Haitians are in the United States "illegally," there is widespread fear that any contact with government agencies will lead to arrest by the Immigration and Naturalization Service, and deportation to Haiti. It is widely appreciated, among Haitians living in the United States, that a positive HIV–1 test is grounds for immediate expulsion. At the time when public health officials were attempting to administer the questionnaire discussed earlier, they must have been concerned about front-page headlines such as "Haitian AIDS victim battles to stay in U.S."[13] For the same reason, one wonders how much the researchers would have learned from their series of questions about illicit drugs.

Many of these research dilemmas were also apparent to the Haitian community leaders who objected to the results of the North American research that led to the inclusion of "Haitian" as a "risk-group." One Haitian researcher and community activist insisted that "there is no way a study (of life-styles) could be done by an American doctor."[14] To whom would he turn to elicit such knowledge? He proposed that Haitian physicians would be better able to extract information about sexual practices from reluctant informants. However, many anthropologists claim that our professional training and extensive fieldwork experience confer a "special understanding" of sexuality that is indispensable to the thorough study of HIV. They do not confer immunity to untruths. On the contrary, "because they never completely become insiders, anthropologists are doubly vulnerable. As 'inside outsiders' and 'outside insiders,' they must contend with a style of lying reserved exclusively for them" (Nachman 1984:538).

Anthropologists were recommended not only for interviewing skills, but also because of an alleged objectivity or neutrality. But how neutral is an anthropologist working for, let us say, a federal bureaucracy? Sponsored research carries its own inherent risks, to which anthropology seems particularly vulnerable (Asad 1975; Berreman 1981). It is for this reason that Hazel Weidman has cautioned against an applied anthropology that leaves unexamined the ways in which the anthropologist's intellectual and moral integrity may be subtly undermined by allegiance to the "system" sponsoring the research. In her view, "the basic 'alienated' stance must be maintained if we are to be truly successful in our applications" (Weidman 1976:108). How best to preserve and to foster the alienated stance in AIDS research, especially when funded by the government, should be a topic of professional debate.

The question of allegiances is not merely a methodological or epistemological problem, but a deeply moral one. In its official statement on ethics, "Principles of Professional Responsibility," the American Anthropological Association reminds its constituents of their responsibilities to those studied, to the public, to the discipline, to students, to sponsors, to the anthropologists' governments, and to host governments. But the anthropologist cannot please everybody, and the "paramount responsibility is to those he (or she) studies. When there is a conflict of interest, these individuals must come first" (cited in Berreman 1981:49). But surely this is too naive a statement, for several reasons. First, most contemporary anthropologists must at least acknowledge that their informants are linked to larger networks of domination and power. These networks may be masked in village settings, but even anthropologists in the most remote hamlets have several "sets" or "classes" of informants. In my work at Do Kay, for example, informants included a young schoolteacher with AIDS, his wife and other family members, his employer, even those accused of bringing his illness upon him. And the village was small enough that Manno's employer was also the ethnographer's host and the person most committed to assuring the continuity of the sick man's medical care. My chief research assistant was a former student of Manno's, and a distant relative of his wife. Alourdes worked in the same school as her husband; one of those accused of killing Manno was her father's brother's daughter and the sister of one of my coworkers and informants; another was more distantly related to Alourdes, but was a trusted key informant with whom I had worked for years. Not all of these informants may have equal claim to the allegiance of the anthropologist.

Issues of confidentiality so central to medicine are not substantially different for the anthropologist. Research that involves persons already exposed to HIV relies on knowledge of laboratory data. In parts of the United States, laws have been enacted to protect the right of those tested to determine who shall have access to the results.[15] In most places in which anthropologists work, however, no such laws exist. How might anthropologists avoid taking advantage of easy access to potentially damaging data? Other questions are equally unexamined. Many anthropologists rely on the help of paid assistants; virtually all of us rely on dependable friends ("key informants") who can be counted on when attempting to unravel a confusing event or interview. If the material collected was recorded on magnetic tape, who helped to transcribe the interviews? Who was privy to the ethnographer's notes?

These dilemmas speak to the need to infuse both our ethical statements and our research with a sensibility to the dynamics of power, whether exercised locally or internationally, nakedly or subtly, directly or indirectly, immediately or with delay. Surely anthropology's pretensions to value-free science or to neutrality have been long ago put to rest. Our undertaking entails responsibilities. But our obligations are neither those of the CDC, nor of any other bureaucracy charged with "protecting the health of the population." Our obligations are also not those of the virologist seeking to develop an anti-HIV vaccine or of the clinician, whose primary responsibilities can justifiably be said to be to his or her patient. Nor are they those of the historian who will one day chart the history of this disease without incurring a debt to living informants.

As HIV "moves along the fault lines of our society" (Bateson and Goldsby 1988:2), it becomes, increasingly, a disease of the disadvantaged. In a discipline that has usually "studied down," taking advantage of the knowledge/power dialectic it is so reluctant to acknowledge, the disempowered should be our natural allies.

## CONCLUSION

"The survival of a nation, of civilized society, of the world itself is said to be at stake—claims that are a familiar part of building a case for repression" (Sontag 1988:85). The AIDS pandemic presents unique challenges to the discipline of anthropology. Because the virus is usually transmitted through intimate contact, because anthropologists *do* have intimate knowledge of the people they study, it may be true, as has so often been claimed, that we have a special role to play in addressing the spread of HIV. But in our eagerness to fight the good fight, anthropology should not forget its often disturbing record on the sharing of special knowledge, its troubled history of collaboration with national and colonial bureaucracies, the mixed fortunes of applied anthropology, its sluggishness in facing the moral dilemmas native to our undertaking in a world in which power is so unevenly distributed. We should not leave unchallenged the messianic optimism of colleagues who predict harmonious and fruitful collaboration with those charged with curbing the spread of HIV.

I believe that careful consideration of topics discussed above will lead anthropologists to the conclusion that, yes, there are ways to share our special knowledge. But how? when? and with whom? In what other ways might we make morally sound contributions to efforts to alleviate the suffering caused by HIV? The manner in which anthropologists participate in "the fight against AIDS" is critical. Given the dim prospects for a vaccine in the near future, and the even dimmer prospects for a cure, it seems safe to say that the anthropological study of HIV poses ethical problems that are unlikely to disappear. To continue to scant this debate by dismissing it as paranoid or obscuring would be lethal to anthropological investigations of AIDS. For wherever AIDS has surfaced, we have seen, accusation has not been far behind. Let us engage these issues before we ourselves are accused of exploiting inequality and anxiety to enhance the status of the already empowered.

## NOTES

I am grateful to Douglas A. Feldman, Arthur Kleinman, Steven Nachman, Jeffrey Parsonnet, and Haun Saussy for their comments on drafts of this chapter. A special debt is owed to Marie-Marcelle Deschamps, a talented and committed physician, and to my Haitian hosts and coworkers, who prefer to be unnamed.

1. Reported in the *Miami Herald*, August 20, 1983, p. 1B.

2. Cited in the *Miami News*, December 2, 1982, p. 8A.

3. It may interest proponents of exotic etiologies that the authors of the only controlled study for risk factors for AIDS among Haitians in the United States reached the following conclusion: "Folklore rituals have been suggested as potential risk factors for HTLV-III/LAV transmission in Haiti. Our data do not support this hypothesis" (Collaborative Study Group of AIDS in Haitian-Americans 1987:638).

4. Nachman and Dreyfuss (1986:33) conclude that "one might at least charge the CDC with poor judgment in treating AIDS as no more than a medical issue and ignoring its social, economic, political, moral and other dimensions. By ignoring these, health officials have seriously hurt the Haitian community. A similar charge can be leveled against medical researchers and clinicians who assume that their scientific and medical priorities are shared by members of the nonmedical community."

5. An assertion countered by Moore and LeBaron (1986:85,88), who not only suggest

that "Gay tourists . . . likely did not bring the disease to Haiti," but that "HTLV-III may have possibly come to Africa with Haitian elites, and in AIDS we may be seeing the spread of a New World disease."

6. The theories that describe Haiti as a "gay Mecca" (e.g., Moore and LeBaron 1986) and those that suggest that homosexuality is particularly stigmatized in Haiti have been questioned, and I believe rightly so, by Murray (1987).

7. Cited in the front page of the *New York Times*, July 31, 1983.

8. Cited in ibid., p. 50.

9. All informants' names are pseudonyms, as are "Do Kay" and "Ba Kay." Other geographical designations are as cited.

10. Although reiteration by no means ensures truthfulness, it should be noted that Manno gave me identical accounts on three different occasions.

11. Cited in *Life*, August 1987, p. 62.

12. From the *Miami News*, August 10, 1983, p. 1.

13. From the *Miami News*, November 1, 1986. The man, who was being held in the INS detention center in South Dade County, was to be deported on charges of drug trafficking.

14. Dr. Jean Claude Desgranges, cited on p. 2A of the May 24, 1983 edition of the *Miami News*.

15. It should be noted, however, that the majority of the legislation advanced in the late 1980's was to *undermine* the rights of those infected with HIV. In most cases, these bills have not been enacted as law.

## REFERENCES

Albert, Edward. 1986. Illness and Deviance: The Response of the Press to AIDS. In *The Social Dimensions of AIDS: Method and Theory*, pp. 163–78. Douglas Feldman and Thomas Johnson, eds. New York: Praeger.

Asad, Talal. 1975. Introduction to *Anthropology and the Colonial Encounter*, pp. 9–19. Talal Asad, ed. London: Ithaca Press.

Bateson, Mary Catherine, and Richard Goldsby. 1988. *Thinking AIDS: The Social Response to the Biological Threat*. Reading, MA: Addison-Wesley.

Berreman, Gerald. 1981. *The Politics of Truth: Essays in Critical Anthropology*. New Delhi: South Asian Publishers.

Casper, Virginia. 1986. AIDS: A Psychosocial Perspective. In *The Social Dimensions of AIDS: Method and Theory*, pp. 197–209. Douglas Feldman and Thomas Johnson, eds., New York: Praeger.

Centers for Disease Control. 1982. Opportunistic infections and Kaposi's sarcoma among Haitians in the United States. *Morbidity and Mortality Weekly Report* 31:353–54, 360–61.

Chaze, William. 1983. In Haiti, a view of life at the bottom. *US News and World Report* 95(18):41–42.

Chen, Kwan-Hwa, and Gerald Murray. 1976. Truths and Untruths in Village Haiti: An Experiment in Third World Survey Research. In *Culture, Natality, and Family Planning*, pp. 241–62. John Marshall and Steven Polgar, eds. Chapel Hill, NC: University of North Carolina Press.

Collaborative Study Group of AIDS in Haitian-Americans. 1987. Risk factors for AIDS among Haitians residing the United States: Evidence of heterosexual transmission. *Journal of the American Medical Association* 257(5):635–39.

Ernst, P., Chen, M. F., Wang, N. S., and M. Cosio. 1983. Symbiosis of *Pneumocystis carinii* and cytomegalovirus in a case of fatal pneumonia. *Canadian Medical Association Journal* 128:1089–92.

Farmer, Paul, and Arthur Kleinman. 1989. AIDS as Human Suffering. *Daedalus*: Vol. 118(2):135–60.

Gilman, Sander. 1988. AIDS and Syphilis: The Iconography of Disease. In *AIDS: Cultural Analysis/Cultural Activism*, pp. 87–107. Douglas Crimp, ed. Cambridge, MA: MIT Press.

Greenfield, W. R. 1986. Night of the Living Dead II: Slow virus encephalopathies and AIDS: Do necromantic zombiists transmit HTLV-III/LAV during voodooistic rituals? *Journal of the American Medical Association* 256:2199–2200.

Landesman, Sheldon. 1983. The Haitian Connection. In *The AIDS Epidemic*, pp. 28–40. Kevin Cahill, ed. New York: St. Martin's Press.

Laverdiere, Michel, Tremblay, Jacques, Lavellee, Rene, Bonny, Yvette Lacombe, Michel, Boileau, Jacques, Lachapelle, Jacques, and Christian Lamoreaux. 1983. AIDS in Haitian immigrants and a Caucasian woman closely associated with Haitians. *Canadian Medical Association Journal* 129:1209–12.

LeBlanc, Robert, Simard, Marie, Flegel, Kenneth and Nobert Gilmore. 1983. Opportunistic infections and acquired cellular immune deficiency among Haitian immigrants in Montreal. *Canadian Medical Association Journal* 129:1205–9.

Liautaud, B., Laroche, D., Duvivier, Jr., and C. Pean-Guichard. 1982. Le sarcome de Kaposi (maladie de Kaposi) est-il frequent en Haiti? Presented at the 18eme Congres des medecins francophones de l'hemisphere americain. Port-au-Prince, Haiti.

Moore, Alexander, and Ronald LeBaron. 1986. The Case for a Haitian Origin of the AIDS Epidemic. In *The Social Dimensions of AIDS: Method and Theory*, pp. 77–93. Douglas A. Feldman and Thomas Johnson, eds. New York: Praeger.

Murray, Stephen. 1986. A Note on Haitian Tolerance of Homosexuality. In *Male Homosexuality in Central and South America*, pp. 92–100. Stephen Murray, ed. Gai Saber Monograph 5.

Nachman, Steven. 1984. Lies my informants told me. *Journal of Anthropological Research* 40:537–55.

Nachman, Steven, and Ginette Dreyfuss. 1986. Haitians and AIDS in South Florida. *Medical Anthropology Quarterly* 17(2):32–33.

Pape, Jean, et al. 1983. Characteristics of the Acquired Immunodeficiency Syndrome (AIDS) in Haiti. *The New England Journal of Medicine* 309(16):945–49.

———. 1985. The Acquired Immunodeficiency Syndrome in Haiti. *Annals of Internal Medicine* 103:674–78.

———. 1987. Epidemiologie de l'Infection HIV en Haiti. *Medica* 2:28–30.

Pape, J. W., Liautaud, B., Thomas, F., Mathurin, J-R., Saint-Amand, M-M., Boncy, M., Pean, V., Verdier, R-I., Deschamps, M-M., and Z. D. Johnson. 1986. Risk factors associated with AIDS in Haiti. *American Journal of Medical Sciences* 29(1):4–7.

Pitchenik, Arthur. 1984. Tuberculosis, Atypical mycobacteria, and AIDS among Haitian and non-Haitian patients in South Florida. *Annals of Internal Medicine* 101:641–45.

Pitchenik, Arthur, Fischl, Margaret, Dickenson, Gordon, Becker, Daniel, Fournier, Arthur, O'Connell, Mark, Colton, Robert, and Thomas Spira. 1983. Opportunistic infections and Kaposi's sarcoma among Haitians: Evidence of a new acquired immunodeficiency state. *Annals of Internal Medicine* 98(3):277–84.

Sabatier, Renee. 1988. *Blaming Others: Prejudice, Race and Worldwide AIDS.* Philadelphia: New Society Publishers.

Scheper-Hughes, Nancy. 1987. The best of two worlds, the worst of two worlds: Reflections on culture and field work among the rural Irish and Pueblo Indians. *Comparative Studies in Society and History* 29(1):56–75.

Sencer, David. 1983. Tracking a Local Outbreak. In *The AIDS Epidemic*, pp. 18–27. Kevin Cahill, ed. New York: St. Martin's Press.

Siegal, Frederick, and Marta Siegal. 1983. *AIDS: The Medical Mystery.* New York: Grove Press.

Smith, Helen. 1983. AIDS: The Haitian connection. *MD* (December):46–52.

Sontag, Susan. 1988. *AIDS and Its Metaphors.* New York: Farrar, Straus & Giroux.

Viera, Jeffrey. 1985. The Haitian Link. In *Understanding AIDS: A Comprehensive Guide.* V. Gong, ed. New Brunswick, NJ: Rutgers.

Viera, J., Frank, E., Spira, T. J., and S. H. Landesman. 1983. Acquired immune deficiency in Haitians: Opportunistic infections in previously healthy Haitian immigrants. *New England Journal of Medicine* 308:125–29.

Weidman, Hazel. 1976. In Praise of the Double Bind Inherent in Anthropological Application. In *Do Applied Anthropologists Apply Anthropology?* Michael Angrosino, ed. Athens, GA: Southern Anthropological Society.

Whitmore, George. 1988. *Someone Was Here: Profiles in the AIDS Epidemic.* New York: New American Library.

# Chapter Seven

## Prostitute Women and the Ideology of Work in London

### Sophie Day

## INTRODUCTION

Research was conducted beginning in August 1986 at the Praed Street Clinic, St. Mary's Hospital, London to look at the relationships between life-style and sexually transmitted infections in a cohort of prostitute women. Prostitution is defined as the exchange of sex for money and/or drugs. A structured questionnaire including sections on social background, work practices, past medical history, and other aspects of life-style is administered where possible on the first visit to the clinic. Subsequent interviews are focused upon a "seven-day recall," relating to the past week's sexual history. However, these later interviews are comparatively informal and unstructured. Records are kept of all interviews and 10 percent of them are taped and transcribed in full. Information collected in the structured questionnaire is checked against information collected over time and by different methods. Women are screened for common genital pathogens at every visit and serology is taken, with consent, every six months. Women are encouraged to attend regularly, ideally monthly, and the provision of appropriate services seems to have promoted re-attendance. In addition to screening and health information, participants are offered treatment for infections by a physician, counseling, and referrals to other health workers where appropriate. These services have been developed as a result of suggestions made by these women.

By the end of 1987, 7 of 112 women recruited had attended only once and had not been seen again during the last six months of the year. These women were assumed to have dropped out of the study. Eighty percent of the cohort were screened for HIV–1 together with a number of other clinic attenders. Three of 130 (2 percent) women prostitutes tested at the clinic are HIV–1 seropositive. Two have shared equipment for injecting drugs, one seems to have been infected through sex with her boyfriend, who was already seropositive.

The cohort includes women working in diverse ways: meeting clients on the streets, in saunas and massage parlors, clubs and hotels, escort agencies, madams, brothels, apartments, and privately. The only large groups of women recruited by the end of 1987 were those who met clients on the streets, through escort agencies, and privately.[1]

This chapter is about the organization of work among prostitutes in which context, it is maintained, discussions of HIV or indeed other infections should be located. It is focused upon common features in the cohort and not upon the many differences among women with regard to working practices, sexuality, or drug use. It would be possible simply to present data on sexually transmitted infections, but these data would not provide much understanding or predictive value on their own. For example, 80 percent of the prostitute women in the cohort now insist that all their clients use condoms; 20 percent do not. These figures do not explain which prostitutes will use condoms, nor why some of those will still acquire sexually transmitted infections. HIV affects people in the course of their lives and its transmission can only be understood when it is also known why, for example, women insist on prophylaxis in the first place and why they have their clients and private partners wear condoms on some occasions and not others—in sum, how they organize their lives.

This chapter, therefore, is an ethnography of work during a period of growing concern with AIDS.[2] Research on prostitutes is often seen to be titillating because of the content of work, "sex for sale," but what is less often appreciated is the preoccupation with work itself. Prostitution is no less fascinating for the student of economics than for the student of sexuality. All the data derive from interviews in the clinic and it should be emphasized that these cannot necessarily be generalized to other London prostitutes, let alone to those working in other areas.

## WORKING GIRLS

Prostitution is very often described as the oldest profession, in such a way that "oldest" acts as a qualifier suggesting that the work both is, and is not, a profession. It is important to appreciate that prostitute women in London present themselves as "business girls" or "working girls," who do business, complain about the lack of business, and are continually on the "look out" for better business. They describe the exchange of sex for money as work and they repudiate any statement that implies it is not. Women also describe themselves as "prostitutes." Occasionally, there is an admission that, even though prostitution is work, it is a rather exceptional kind of work. Women sometimes say that they are "on the game" or they describe non-prostitutes as "straight." Sometimes, they call themselves "whores" or "hookers." Note the following conversation with Julia[3], a woman from the Midlands in her mid-twenties, who turns down most of the work offered her by the agencies:

*Julia*: I hate that word (prostitute).

*Interviewer*: Some people say business girls.

*Julia*: That's even worse. I'm a worker.

*Interviewer*: Yes. Lots of people describe themselves as working girls.

*Julia*: No. I'm just a worker. You hear hooker sometimes. Some of the older ones, who've been around for a while, they call themselves hookers. I'm not working. I'm a worker.

One woman, June, says:

*June*: I work three days a week (in a sauna) at the moment. There's a possibility of a fourth, on Sunday. But that still leaves me sitting on my butt three days a week. I might try the agency again, just one case (client) a day would help.

*Interviewer*: That would give you a seven-day week.

*June*: Well, at least it would keep the money coming through the bank.

June is a Londoner with extensive experience in saunas, apartments, and escort agencies. Like almost every other woman I have met who has been working for more than a few months, she adds that business is bad. It is much worse in 1987 than it was a year before. Perhaps it is the AIDS scare, the number of young girls flooding the market, or, at the appropriate times: Ramadan, some crisis in the Middle East, the exchange rate, or the Libyan bombings. Prostitution in London involves foreign clients as much as nationals and so women correspondingly stress international affairs in describing the state of business. Indeed, they see their work as a highly sensitive indicator of fluctuations in the money supply or the political status quo. Although it is clear that certain sectors in prostitution have been adversely affected by developments in the last few years, such as the amount of Middle Eastern money in London, there is no reason to suppose that the overall volume of work or money has declined. Rather, it seems that those who present themselves as "business girls" and "working girls" are preoccupied with the state of the market. Such comments are often followed by a series of probing questions and I am seen as a potential consultant who is likely to know who is making the money, where and how.

Like those with small businesses the world over, prostitutes almost always say that business is bad. Maureen, an erstwhile hairdresser from Yorkshire, describes how she then goes about looking for work. I had just been asked for advice on her various options:

I've been invited to Sweden next week to act in a pornographic movie. They're offering me 22,000 [pounds sterling] for six weeks. I'm really worried about AIDS. I definitely won't be able to use durex [condom] there and I can't decide whether to go or not.

Laura, who's drawing up my contracts, is going to make six grand [6,000] out of it. . . . There is a second alternative . . . I've been asked to do soft porn pictures for 5,000 over four to six weeks. So, I might do that if I decide not to do the movie.

If I got the 22,000, I probably wouldn't have to work again or only with regulars who are really safe. Then I could set up a small business. I really don't like working.

Two months later, Maureen returned. She had not done the film or the photos. She said:

I don't know how it all fell through. I was really desperate. There was no work. . . . So, I agreed to go to Bahrain with this girl. She said she'd earned 19 grand [19,000 pounds sterling] but she didn't tell me it was four years ago and it took four months. It was terrible. We worked in a flat [apartment] and got ripped off. I had to work twelve to twelve and there was nothing to do, cooped up in the flat with no one to talk to. I left after a week and I lost money.

I'm desperate for property, for a mortgage. There are such high overheads on the flat and, because I'm not from here, I can't get housing. I don't want a flat to live in. I couldn't afford to do that. But to rent out. I can't even manage a down payment at the moment. So, I'm thinking of going to Dubai with another friend who worked there last summer. I trust her. I'm not sure what the set-up is, but you stay in a hotel so you can do what you like; you're your own boss. The good thing would be, first, I'd get some money, but then I'll also pick up private references for when they come through London for two weeks without their wives and I'll get commission, like a madam, by sending them on. So, I could build up a business by making a trip to the Middle East.

These comments provide good examples of the way London prostitutes talk about "business." Many are prepared to move to where the money is, either long-term—15 of the women we see are from other countries—and short-term, in the way Maureen describes.

This common preoccupation with work is all the more striking as it is set against a background of great diversity. Maureen works for agencies and madams as well as privately, while June works at a sauna. Maureen sees herself as an entrepreneur who will, with luck, set up a "small business" and "build up a business" while June just puts in the hours, earning more money than she could in another service job but doing basically the same kind of thing, as she sees it. Indeed, when June stresses the everyday nature of her work, she describes herself as a "social worker" who performs an essential service. She repeats the common view that men have "instinctive" aggressive appetites that must be satisfied: If they cannot pay prostitutes for sex, they will rape other women. Similar arguments are put forward by prostitutes about marriage: If men could not visit prostitutes, they would take it out on their wives, or they would have messy affairs that would ruin their marriages.

Laura came to London from a town in the south of the country over two years ago because she was no longer able to support herself on a clerical salary. She works for agencies, madams, and on her own. Laura also emphasizes her role as "social worker" when she says that she relieves men of their sexual appetites though she acts primarily as a companion or hostess. "My job, as far as I can see it, is to be the perfect hostess, very jolly company, very chatty. As you can tell, I laugh a lot. I keep them happy. My job when I get back is just to relieve them, that's all. As far as I'm concerned, that's it." Such arguments do not only seek to establish prostitution as work, but as *essential* work or service.

All of these women stress the everyday nature of their work and they try to infuse prostitution with everyday notions such as skill, boredom, routine, pay, or control over the work process. Caroline, for example, speaks of dissociation from work. She initially came to the clinic for about six months when she was 17 years old, having moved to London from Yorkshire. She works on the streets:

When I get into the area of the beat [a street area where prostitutes work], I switch off my body and my mind. I'm very alert to everything, very sharp and irritable. I'm usually in a car and I'm in and out like a zombie. I sit in the back and, before I do anything, I get them to pay cash, in English money.

Caroline insists that prostitution is work, reserved for work hours and workplaces. The process of "switching off" that she describes is evocative of labor in other contexts.[4] Another prostitute who works privately also insists that what she does is work but she speaks of a very different aspect, skill. She says that she will have to find some "sex work" because she has such a huge overdraft but, this time, she will only do lesbian scenes: "There will be no fucking. I'll work out what they want ahead of time with a friend. It's much more skilled and you have much more control over what happens." A woman who works at an exclusive gentleman's health club stresses the importance of experience in the job. She has worked at this club for five years:

They pretend they don't know about it. So you give a massage and then whatever else they want. But, you can't ask for money first. It's a tip. Sometimes, they just walk out without paying and there's nothing you can do. But, I've learned to agree to a price first. I just tell them the minimum. If the management found out, I'd be fired. So all the clients try and get the new girls. They know they won't have to pay. That's why I'm thinking of trying another place.

The prostitutes who visit the clinic come from 11 different countries and a wide range of workplaces and social classes. They rarely work together; indeed, one of the more important aspects of prostitution in London concerns an en-forced isolation at the workplace.[5] The universal concern to stress prostitution as a form of work carries all the more significance against this background.

The quality of these assertions might be explored further as part of an op-positional stance that sets itself against popular views of prostitution. These dwell in some wonder upon the historicity of "the oldest profession" and upon the content of work, sex for sale, rather than its organization. Prostitutes also clearly have their doubts. A repeated insistence upon the perfectly ordinary nature of the work often seems to represent an attempt to persuade the worker herself of the truth of this assertion. Julia, for example, who describes herself above as a "worker," spent the next half hour of that interview telling me how normal she was and how normal she wanted to be. She appealed to a popular image of reasonable behavior as she said: "I could be chatting happily to an old woman on the bus. But, if she knew, she'd move her seat, wouldn't she." At times, prostitutes also turn toward the majority view and their counter-ideology falters. It seems that the exchange of sex for money is not exactly work and not perhaps part of mainstream British culture.

In the face of such doubts, it is not surprising that prostitutes try to strengthen their own position. The rest of this chapter explores one aspect of their focus on work: its hoped-for autonomy. In order for prostitution to look like work, it must exist separately from all that is not work. A great deal of effort is expended in circumscribing, limiting, and demarcating work from what prostitutes consider to be their private selves and their true personhood.

At first sight, this division looks straightforward, simple to construct and also to maintain. A prostitute creates distinctions with her body so that work involves very little physical contact in contrast to private sexual contacts. Thus, condoms are worn at work and only certain types of sex are acceptable while sex outside work involves neither physical barriers nor forbidden zones. Prostitutes divide their social world similarly so that clients belong to a world of work governed by a market morality while private life is reserved for the family and a kinship morality; the perspective of money is thereby contrasted with that of love.

These divisions are described later in this chapter. In addition, it will be seen that the two worlds can scarcely be kept apart. There is the boyfriend who lives off a woman's earnings. Women in the cohort often described past but not current boyfriends of this kind as pimps, yet they always found it hard to draw a clear distinction between the two. There is the regular client who provides substantial financial support and who falls in love with a woman. There may be a supportive network of friends who identify with a subculture and continually mix work with private concerns. There is also the broken condom which allows their clients' semen to enter (and implicitly violate) the prostitute's body. London prostitutes in the cohort find that their private lives are constantly on the point of dissolving into work.

## DIVISIONS OF THE BODY

Prostitute women attempt to minimize all contact with clients so as to preserve themselves for their private partners of choice. Some prostitutes stress the preliminary companionship and downplay the actual sex. Women such as Laura manage to see themselves as companions who spend just a few minutes at the end of an evening having sex with or masturbating their clients. Many sauna workers and an increasing number of escort and private workers describe how they avoid sex altogether. It is not always clear whether "sex" then means any sexual contact or just penetrative intercourse (i.e., vaginal, oral, or anal sex). A number of sauna workers describe themselves as "ex-prostitutes," who have given up selling sex although they continue to masturbate their clients for money. Thus, one sauna worker says that she now only sells "hand relief" or masturbation: "Prostitution is just actual intercourse."

A number of women are now encouraging similar activities where clients do not penetrate the body itself; for example, they offer "breast relief," where a client masturbates between a woman's breasts. Some women avoid physical contact with their clients altogether by selling a variety of fantasies; they have "make-believe scenes" with other women in front of a client and practice domination. This specialized work is thought to pose less of a threat to the person because the client is kept outside the body.

Where sexual penetration becomes inevitable, a number of further techniques are described which keep the client away and the prostitute detached. Women like Caroline speak of switching off. The type of sexual encounter is restricted and, perhaps most important, latex barriers (condoms and caps or diaphragms) are used. Caroline's comments are typical:

I see two or three punters [clients] a night. I won't kiss them. With people I've known [for the past four months] . . . then I will. Oral sex is vile. They think you're enjoying it. But, with straight sex, you can lie there like a sack of potatoes. I always use a sheath (condom). I'd commit suicide if I didn't.

Whatever the differences among prostitutes in the cohort, all are preoccupied with keeping their distance. When sex occurs, it is carefully controlled, critically through the use of condoms. Caroline says she would commit suicide without a condom. Laura uses a diaphraghm, a spermicidal pessary, spermicide, and a condom as well as oral contraceptives. Recently, when she was trying to get pregnant and had stopped taking oral contraceptives, she became very worried about the possibility of impregnation by clients. Another participant in the study said that she always puts two condoms on clients; she says they never notice. Now, however, she is seriously considering using three in order to protect herself from AIDS.

Women say that semen is dirty; it is the semen as well as any organisms it might carry that are rejected. However, it seems that only clients have dirty semen and it is the substances associated with work that must be kept outside the body. Given these attitudes, it would be surprising to find that the use of prophylaxis is a new phenomenon among London prostitutes. Condom use in 46 prostitutes who attended the clinic regularly until May 1987 was assessed. Twenty-five of them (54 percent) reported condom use all the time with their clients at their first visit to the clinic. By May 1987, 13 more women were using condoms in this way and so a total of 83 percent were reporting condom use for every client contact. Although women are better protected than they were, because of the fear of AIDS, it is important to realize that there always has been a general desire to keep clients' semen out of the body.

If women turn work into a distinctive domain by means of a battery of protective devices, they also restrict permissible types of sex with clients. As Caroline says, "oral sex is vile" but vaginal sex is alright because "you can lie there like a sack of potatoes." Laura too speaks of "straight sex": ". . . I can lie back and think of England or write shopping lists." Few women currently sell anal sex largely because of its association with gay male sex which is now condemned as "dirty." Women said of the anus, "it's not made for that," and several went into details about how the vagina was self-cleansing unlike the anus. Sex through "the back," said some, was "unnatural." Interestingly, while the risks of HIV from anal sex may indeed be higher than vaginal intercourse, the women are also selling less oral sex and clients usually wear condoms during oral intercourse.

In this way, women in London are increasingly left with vaginal intercourse.[6] First, it is thought to be "natural"—it is described as "straight sex" and thereby associated with non-prostitute women. Second, it is "down there." It seems that prostitute women are making the same kinds of bodily discriminations as other groups (see, for example, Sutherland 1975) so that sex "down there" comes to belong to work; it can be sold and thereby alienated from the person, while sex that involves the upper part of the body is increasingly saved for the self and for domestic life. In other words, attempts are made to lessen the intrusion of work into the private person. Vaginal sex is assumed to be the most popular activity with clients in most contexts and prostitutes are prepared to treat the vagina as a commodity at work. However, they resist this process with respect to any other parts of their bodies. Thus, as Caroline says, there is no kissing. Oral sex involves the (private) mouth and so, today, it is avoided or realigned with the public domain by means of condoms. The parts of the body that can be hired out are those involved in "straight sex" and, in the current climate, this kind of sale is seen to be less risky.

The body is used in these ways to set up an autonomous working environment. Sex at home should be easily demarcated. Caroline takes a more extreme position than most but expresses a common sentiment, since she distinguishes sex at work from love at home.

My Christmas is July 23, Haile Selassie's birthday [she is a white Rastafarian.] I'm very strict. I read the Bible every day. Your body is your temple. I'm abusing it as a prostitute. I pray a lot. I don't go to church, and I don't eat pig. God is inside me. Your body is your church. I don't believe in sex, only in making love.

At every visit, prostitutes are asked about their sexual activities over the previous week. One question concerns "the last time you had sexual intercourse—that is, penetration." Julia's answer never seemed to fit with the details that she gave later about her work and her boyfriend. During the course of a particular interview, I asked, "Was that with your boyfriend or a client?" She said, "What?" I explained what I had meant. After what seemed to be a long pause, she realized that this question applied both to work and to her personal life. She reprimanded me, "I call work 'work.' That's all it is. I've always told you about my boyfriend when you asked that."

This division is buttressed by means of the use of prophylaxis at work but *not* at home. Only three women (3 percent) reported any condom use with their boyfriends and, for two of them, condoms were intended only to prevent pregnancy. Other women were horrified at the thought of using anything with their private (nonpaying) partners. In most cases, they said it would simply finish the relationship. Maureen, for example said, "We have a very good sex life. It would be spoiled if he wore a sheath (condom). We would be finished." Another woman sums it up, "I don't want strangers' semen inside. I only drop the barrier with someone I really love." And Rachel adds, "How could I? He would be like a client. It's different for people who don't work" (i.e., sell sex).

Sex with a boyfriend or husband is also linked to procreation, while work must never lead to children. Contraception is often distinguished from protection and specified as an intrauterine device (IUD)—"coil," or oral contraceptive—"the pill." One woman had been sterilized. Another deals with her worries about AIDS in an elaborate fashion. To make sure that she is protected at every contact with a client, she has stopped taking the pill. She feels that the double risk, of infection and conception, will ensure that she never forgets to make her clients wear condoms. Nowadays, then, the condom serves her as a contraceptive as well as a protective device. For most of the women, this area of overlap occurs only when they are trying to get pregnant. The practicalities of achieving pregnancy at home while avoiding it at work are often complicated and accompanied by some anxiety about burst condoms and, in the event of pregnancy, paternity. The use of contraception extends bodily divisions between work and private life.

Furthermore, the pleasures of sex at home might involve any part of the body. A number of women say that they have oral sex with their boyfriends but never at work. Interestingly, this is described as the only type of private sex for two of the women in the study. A few sheepishly admit to anal sex after a few interviews, but only at home. When asked about work, they explain how difficult this would be because clients would hurt you; boyfriends can be trusted. Moreover, they say, clients who want anal sex are bound to be bisexuals and, therefore, at risk for AIDS.

All these bodily divisions seem to be straightforward. Women avoid physical contact with clients as much as possible; they clothe the penis in latex and they restrict it to the bottom half of the body. Contraception is used. Barriers are dropped, however, with boyfriends. Types of sex are not restricted. These divisions are general but they are not universal. A number of other physical divisions may be associated with what, it is hoped, will prove to be an adequate demarcation of work.

Some women refuse to have sex at all in their private lives. Two-thirds of the women seen by May 1987 had boyfriends or husbands (52/77) but about half of the one-third who did not described this as a deliberate strategy. One woman explains:

I'm all on my own. I can't even have a dog. There's a girl who sometimes has to leave her dog locked inside without food for two days when she's doing a job. I couldn't have a boyfriend in this business. First, I'm up and about at all hours; second, what about the money? Girls with boyfriends, they have more problems than me.

Three women describe themselves as lesbians. They see men at work and women at home. All three women find it easier to separate their working lives from their home life because of this categorical gender distinction. Finally, a majority of those with boyfriends/husbands make a further distinction based on color. These predominantly white prostitutes have black boyfriends and white clients. In fact, the distinction may be more finely drawn. Some women say they avoid clients from the Caribbean, by which they generally refer to British nationals, for fear of violence, but they will accept Africans. At least, they would if they could distinguish the two populations at first contact. Prostitutes who work in apartments and brothels, as well as some of those who work privately, employ maids to get potential clients. These maids are rarely trusted to distinguish between African and Caribbean clients. The private partners of these women are ethnically Caribbean and British citizens. Three women in the cohort are also ethnically Caribbean.

The distinctions described are clearly also social divisions. In particular, it is suggested that "the boyfriend as pimp" and the "regular client" confound the division between work and personal life so thoroughly that they become intertwined. For the majority of heterosexual women in the cohort, only children seem to offer the possibility of creating two truly autonomous environments. As women make a home around children, they also succeed in setting up a bounded domain of work.

## SOCIAL DIVISION

The previous section has shown how social divisions are created by means of the body, with clients on one side and boyfriends on the other. Divisions based upon money (in contrast to love) and secrecy (with respect to those at home) are equally important in this respect. As women describe how business is negotiated so that it becomes part of a clearly demarcated working life, they talk not just of how they use their bodies but also of money. As they outline the strict guidelines about permissible behavior, they talk especially about receiving their money beforehand and timing an encounter in terms of material benefit. Thus, Laura says that she will only stay half an hour if she is not being taken out to dinner. The minimum booking fee is two hours (from an agency) and she describes the other hour and a half as profit. Most of the women describe time as money. Mary is nearly 40 years of age and she came to England from southern Europe over 15 years ago. She works privately in an apartment that she owns. She talks of lost rather than gained time with her "sugar daddy," (i.e., an established client who sees himself as a boyfriend):

He gives me 200 pounds [sterling]. It's spending money. It can be a holiday with the pool and the sun [in Marbella] but look at what I lost. Nearly a week. Roger [the pseudonym of a client] disappeared, I haven't seen him since. The others went to Susan [a friend who works with Mary]. I lost nearly a thousand pounds [sterling]. I can't afford to go again. He should give me more, but he doesn't know.

Caroline requests her money beforehand in British cash. Although many women now accept checks and credit cards, and although fewer now insist upon British notes which are counted out before any further exchange, it is still the money transaction that defines work. Particular sexual services and time are calculated in terms of money. The private sphere ought to exclude this emphasis on money and base itself upon ties of love and affection. London prostitutes particularly stress the personal choice of friends and sexual partners.

Secrecy creates a further barrier. On the whole, people in one's private life do not usually know about one's work. Only three of the women I know have told their mothers about their work. Most are less concerned about the rest of their families. One woman, Caroline, said that what she liked least about prostitution " . . . is lying to my mum and dad and the rest [of the family] in Yorkshire. Perhaps, I will just work one or two nights for clothes and do a day job for the rest [of the money I need]. Social [social security] will pay for the flat." Caroline, however, was in a juvenile court for soliciting a year ago and, though there were times in London when her mother did not seem to know what she was doing, Caroline could not separate her work sufficiently from her family to be able to maintain the fiction that she was working as an assistant at a jewelry shop.

None of the women tell their children about their work. Indeed, the difficulties they have in keeping their work to themselves as children grow up provide one of the major motivations for changing or stopping work. Ten women in the cohort have children and eight of the ten live with their children. Mary, the woman from southern Europe, has an 11-year-old son whom she has just sent to boarding school:

I'm very lonely. Now that Simon's [a pseudonym for the son] at school, I should be working but I can't be bothered. . . . I'm having moral problems about it. What if my son found out? I don't care about anyone else, but he really is my friend. I hate lying to him.

Mary is in the middle of a second divorce from her husband, whom she had remarried. He knows something of her work and Mary is currently obsessed with what he might tell their son during the traumas of divorce.

The desire for secrecy extends to the variety of names used by the prostitutes in the study. Many stories that are told become impossible to follow because of the bewildering variety of names that are used. I might be given one name for personal letters, another in the clinic environment, while a third is mentioned incidentally in the course of a story. Someone will describe a phone call that puzzled her because she could not decide whether it was a wrong number or a call from a very old contact using a name that had not been hers for some years. Someone else will tell me a story about her friend, fumbling suddenly as she tries to remember what name I know that woman by. The use of a number of names is clearly related to the desire for confidentiality and it is also related directly to the division that is made between home and work. Mary, for example, tries to create an unambiguous distinction by using one name for work and another at home, with a slight variation on her work name in related areas such as taxation and clinic attendance.

There seem to be two contrasting positions with regard to female friends. Some women prefer non-prostitute ("straight") friends, because they will belong only to the domestic sphere and so it will be easier to keep that sphere separate from the working environment. Others prefer prostitute friends because they can talk about mutual interests. There are extensive personal networks among the women we see, though these are often partially hidden because of the number of names that are used.

Other social divisions are made but, for the present purposes, one last example will show how distinctions remain important to prostitutes even when they are hidden from the people around them. Very few women ever see clients at home. Such men are likely to be private clients who have a woman's home telephone number and who provide her with a dependable source of income. Even when women see these "regulars" at home, they manage to distinguish work and private life by turning a room into a temporary workplace, as one woman describes:

My boyfriend hates it. He says he don't want no punter [client] in his bed. But, it's not my bed. I have three towels. I put one over the pillow, one over the mattress and there's one for him to wash with. Nobody except for clients ever touches those towels and they're even washed separately.

In other words, the bed is transformed into a public place through the addition of towels.

In spite of these emphatic and far-reaching divisions, the barrier between work and home is flimsy and it is always on the point of collapse if not actually falling down. There are two key threats. The first comes from work, not from the casual but from the regular client. The second comes from the private sphere, from the boyfriend.

Regular clients may have privileged types of bodily contact with prostitutes. Mary, for example, has anal sex with one regular. Like many women we see, she does not use condoms consistently with regular clients. Money is frequently evaluated in a very different way from the transactions that occur with casual or new clients. Sometimes, regular clients do not pay; on other occasions, they agree to pay private medical bills or school fees. A woman in the cohort plans to have a thyroid operation and she says one of her regulars will pay. Another woman has to have surgery which will stop her working for six months. Although there will be no medical expenses, she says that a regular client has agreed to pay all her other bills during that period, which will amount to 6,000 pounds sterling.

In all these ways, regulars occupy a "fuzzy" area in between (casual) clients and boyfriends. They attack the division between work and home. However, they do not undermine that barrier as extensively as boyfriends, who threaten to turn what seemed to be a private life into an extension of the workplace.

Women with regular private partners usually support them to a significant extent and they worry about their motives. A private partner who knows about your work is, by definition, a pimp. In law, this is the case but it is also true in a more subtle sense because women can never know that their partners are interested just in their private lives and not their work. They can never know whether the boyfriend is not getting paid twice over, once in cash or more general support and, again, in getting sex for free. One woman explicitly recognized these financial motives and explained that a prostitute uses her pimp in the same way that clients use her: clients buy sex from prostitutes and prostitutes buy sex or companionship from pimps. Boyfriends and husbands can never be insulated from work if they know that their women work as prostitutes and the overlap is expressed largely through the idiom of money which has a tendency to unite the two domains.

London prostitutes are less worried about clients infiltrating their homes than they are about losing their homes and private selves to work. Relations with boyfriends are part of work or it is feared that they will become so. Moreover, relations with families and, generally, friends are unreal because they are based upon a fiction of the working individual who does not sell sex, and they are attenuated in an attempt to maintain this fiction. Prostitutes may fail to set up a domain of work because they cannot build a separate and mutually defining home.

Conception, pregnancy, and motherhood provide a radical solution to this problem. Prostitute women in London exchange sex for money during their working hours; in their private lives they build homes. Heterosexual women retain their true selves and their domestic lives through children.

There seems to be an extraordinary preoccupation with possible infertility among the women I have interviewed. This fear of sterility is a real concern. Laura says,

I've been cleaner since I started working. I use durex (condoms), (contraceptive) pessaries, a sponge and spermicide. Before, I got gonorrhea, trichomonas and chlamydia. It has spread to my tubes. Sometimes, they say, that can make you sterile.

Laura, in fact, became pregnant with the ex-boyfriend. They are friendly once more but, she says, she will never live with him again. She has bought a house close to her parents and she is renting a room to her brother to help pay the mortgage. Meanwhile, she visits London occasionally to see clients. Her plans are to go to college here in London and then teach part-time. Laura's pregnancy has drawn her back to the family fold.

In more general terms, it should be appreciated that the symbolic load attached to motherhood is very great. Adult dependents are seen to share too many qualities with pimps to be able to be moved entirely into the domestic domain. The relationship is tainted by money and cannot be transformed into a purely private one. Children are the only dependents and companions who will not be drawn into the sphere of work even if they are supported through prostitution. Much of the publicity that prostitute women have had published in recent years illustrates this image very clearly. Jaget (1980), for example, portrays prostitutes above all as mothers in a description of a sit-in by French prostitutes in response to ill-treatment by police.

Nuclear families, with the father, mother, and children living together, are rare in the cohort. None of the fourteen women who are pregnant or who have children currently live with the father. The basic family unit is the mother and child. These residential arrangements could be described as matrifocal (see, for example, Hannerz 1969; Smith 1963, 1973) and related to the problems of integrating sex with domestic life.

What then initially looks like a simple opposition between clients and private partners or between work and personal life turns out to be a continuum with casual clients at one extreme and children, or the status of mother, at the other. Neither regular clients nor boyfriends/husbands can be located firmly on just one side of the divide.

## CONCLUSION: RISKS OF HIV TRANSMISSION

Of the three HIV-positive prostitute women, two have been infected through shared equipment for drug use, and one seems to have been infected sexually by her boyfriend, who is also a pimp. Condoms are not worn with boyfriends. It is not known whether these men are at other risk of HIV infection but is is worth noting that women in the cohort consider themselves to be at risk of infections from their boyfriends. Exactly half (26/52) of the women with boyfriends on whom detailed information had been collected by May 1987 said that they *knew* (rather than suspected) that their boyfriends had other sexual partners. It was thought by the women that condoms were not used with these other partners.

Condoms are used with clients in order to protect a sense of personal integrity and to separate work from private life. A further, more general, comment might be made on the symbolic appropriateness of condom use at work. In much of the literature on protection and contraception, devices such as the condom are seen to be non-natural and therefore inappropriate by those who are encouraged to use them (see, for example, MacCormack and Draper 1987:158). Among London prostitutes, the "unnatural" qualities of condoms may be seen in positive terms. They are manufactured in the economic and public domain and they may therefore be particularly appropriate to work processes in contrast to a "natural" sex life at home.

Since condoms provide protection against HIV infection, it is likely that prostitute women in the London cohort will not become infected with HIV from their clients. Similarly, clients may be protected from infection because of condom use. However, women in the cohort continue to be at potential risk from sexual contacts with their private partners. If infected, their future children will also be at risk.

Epidemiologic research has clearly established the risk of HIV transmission associated with shared equipment for injecting drugs among prostitute populations in developed nations (Tirelli 1986; Centers for Disease Control 1987). This chapter has identified another potential route of transmission associated with prostitutes' private, non-paying partners. Only one woman in the cohort seems to have acquired HIV infection in this way to date. However, a continuing study of the organization of prostitution in London confirms the potential importance of this context in the absence of current HIV infection. An anthropological approach has suggested the relevance of aspects of prostitution which are not generally emphasized in the context of HIV transmission. These aspects are not directly concerned with the sale of sex nor are they associated with particularly high rates of partner change. It is suggested that a close focus on the social and cultural context is therefore essential to research on HIV transmission for, as the present example suggests, this focus may anticipate future developments as well as help in the interpretation of current patterns of infection. Moreover, the present example reveals clear priorities for preventive programs. The promotion of universal condom use among prostitutes will depend upon an understanding of the potential significance for HIV transmission of sex outside work. It will depend also upon an understanding of the double significance of the condom, which provides not just a physical barrier to infection but also a symbolic barrier between working and private life. Health programs will then be able to anticipate the difficulties of introducing condoms into the private sexual relationships of London prostitutes. Success will depend at least partly upon the reconstruction of alternative symbolic barriers between different domains of prostitutes' lives.

## NOTES

I would like to acknowledge the AIDS Virus and Education Research Trust which has funded my research project with prostitute women for a three year period, beginning in August, 1986. I am also very grateful to the women cited in this chapter, and to Maurice Bloch, who commented upon an earlier draft of this chapter.

1. Prostitutes who meet clients on the streets may take them to hotels or apartments. They may also solicit in or near hotels. Women who work in saunas, clubs, and escort agencies generally meet clients through a third party such as a manager. Some London agencies are "sit-in": prostitutes sit in the agency during work hours, but most operate by telephone. Prostitutes are available on a certain number during the required period. Madams might be described as unofficial escort agencies who refer clients to prostitutes by telephone. Apartments generally consist of one or more women and maid who admits clients; services are advertised. Brothels might be described as larger apartments though they generally also have a manager, often one of the prostitutes. Women who work privately are referred clients by other prostitutes and other clients.

2. There is a large ethnographic literature on "work." See, for example, Godelier's (1980) programmatic article in the *History Workshop Journal*, articles in S. Wallman (1979) (ed.), *Social Anthropology of Work*, Paul E. Willis's (1983, orig. 1977) *Learning to Labour*, Rosendhal's (1985) *Conflict and Compliance*, and Agar's (1986) *Independents Declared: The Dilemmas of Independent Trucking*.

My emphasis on work is intended, in part, to provide a corrective to biases in previous accounts where prostitutes are seen as "victims" with no control over their occupation and as "deviants." See, for example, Cohen (1980). Bujra makes a similar point when she writes:

It is not easy to find models for an objective sociological analysis of prostitution. Much of the literature on the subject, if not merely descriptive, is charged with a moralistic tone or with psychological insinuations—it sees prostitution as a "social problem," as "deviant behavior," or as an indication of "psychological immaturity." (Bujra 1975:214)

3. Personal names are pseudonyms. Extensive quotations are made verbatim from interviews.

4. One of the best accounts of this process of dissociation can be found in Willis (1977). He describes how working class "lads" deal with the shopfloor in a way that is very similar to the accounts prostitutes give of their work. Willis argues, "Basically this concerns an experiential separation of the inner self from work. Labour power is a kind of barrier to, not an inner connection with, the demands of the world. Satisfaction is not expected in work" (1983:102).

5. The law reinforces isolation in the workplace as women can only work legally alone and they cannot support their adult partners. One prostitute says she will not share with another woman because the other woman could be arrested for being thought to be a madam. Similarly, she does not live with her boyfriend because he would be in danger of being arrested for pimping.

6. Other types of sex are also sold. Clients occasionally perform cunnilingus on prostitutes. Some prostitutes perform active anal sex on clients with a dildo, although they rarely describe this as "anal sex." A condom is generally used on the dildo. Nonpenetrative sex includes a wide range of generally specialized practices, in addition to those mentioned

in the text, including bondage, "watersports" (where the prostitute urinates on a client), dressing up, and other fantasies.

## REFERENCES

Agar, Michael H. 1986. *Independents Declared: The Dilemmas of Independent Trucking.* Smithsonian Series in Ethnographic Inquiry 4. Washington, DC: Smithsonian Institute Press.

Bujra, J. M. 1975. Women "Entrepreneurs" of Early Nairobi. *Canadian Journal of African Studies* 9:213–34.

Centers for Disease Control. 1987. Antibody to human immunodeficiency virus in female prostitutes. *MMWR* 36:157–61.

Godelier, Maurice. 1980. Work and its Representations: A Research Proposal. *History Workshop* 10:164–74.

Hannerz, U. 1969. *Soulside: Inquiries into Ghetto Culture and Community.* New York: Columbia University Press.

Jaget, Claude, ed. 1980 [1975]. *Prostitutes: Our Life.* Translated from the French by Anna Furse, Suzie Fleming, and Ruth Hall. London: Falling Wall Press.

MacCormack, C., and Draper, A. 1987. Social and cognitive aspects of female sexuality in Jamaica. In *The Cultural Construction of Sexuality*, pp. 143–65. Pat Caplan, ed. London: Tavistock Publications.

Rosendhal, Mona. 1985. Conflict and Compliance: Class consciousness among Swedish workers. *Stockholm Studies in Social Anthropology* 14.

Smith, R. T. 1963. Culture and Social Structure in the Caribbean: Some recent work on family and kinship studies. *Comparative Studies in Society and History* 6:24–46.

———. 1973. The Matrifocal Family. In *The Character of Kinship*, pp. 121–44. J. Goody, ed. Cambridge: Cambridge University Press.

Sutherland, Anne. 1975. *Gypsies: The Hidden Americans.* London: Tavistock.

Tirelli, U., Vaccher, E., Sorio, R. et al. 1986. HTLV-III Antibodies in Drug Addicted Prostitutes used by US Soldiers in Italy (letter). *JAMA* 256:711–12.

Wallman, Sandra, ed. 1979. *Social Anthropology of Work.* ASA Monograph 19. London: Academic Press.

Willis, P. E. 1983 [1977]. *Learning to Labour: How Working Class Kids Get Working Class Jobs.* Aldershot: Gower.

# Chapter Eight

## Minority Women and AIDS: Culture, Race, and Gender

### Dooley Worth

Heterosexual AIDS education in the United States is targeted primarily at women, particularly poor black and Latina women who make up 70 percent of female AIDS cases. The effect of AIDS on minority women, and their response to AIDS education, is poorly understood in the absence of examination of the political economies which shape the gender, class, and race relations of individual women's lives and identities, and the specific impact of racial, social, and economic oppression on socialization patterns in minority communities.

In speaking about the socialization of Latina women in the United States, and its impact on cultural expectations, McKenna and Ortiz have noted that, "the notion of choices, and how and why [women] make them is critical" (1988, 67).

Cultural values are the medium through which sexuality, drug use, and disease are interpreted and acted upon. They determine how a woman will conceptualize, define, and label the behavioral choices she will make (Vance 1985, 8).

Culturally determined values influence how individual perceptions of AIDS are selected, how attitudes toward high-risk behavior are formed, how habits that characterize high-risk behavior are developed, and how risk-reduction information will be processed.

Individual behavior choices are poorly understood because there has been a lack of interest in learning how cultural values and expectations are related to socioeconomic survival skills of women in specific minority communities.[1]

Behavioral change (which is correlated to cultural change), cannot be promoted successfully without understanding the structural determinants (i.e., poverty, poor housing, low levels of educational achievement, acculturation pressures, racism, sexism) and their influence on gender behavior, sexuality, drug use, and health behaviors related to the prevention of AIDS.[2]

Examining the relationship between gender behavior, class, and race is essential. Gender relations are among society's most crucial modulators of individual behavior and they dictate not only how women should behave as women, but what their relationship should be to the dominant society (Fox-Genovese 1988, 194).

This chapter draws on studies of the effect of poverty, racism, non-acculturation pressures on the cultural beliefs and expectations of impoverished Puerto Rican and U.S. born (non-Haitian or non-African) black women in New York.[3] It is exploratory in nature, meant to stimulate further discussion of the need for anthropological research to complement epidemiologic studies of the high rate of HIV transmission in minority communities.[4]

Before exploring the impact of poverty, racism, and acculturation pressures on the women and communities most vulnerable to contracting AIDS, it is instructive to look at societal responses to the AIDS epidemic.

## DISEASE AND "OTHERNESS"

Throughout Western history disease has been associated with isolation as social opposition is created between the healthy (us) and the diseased (them). Primitive tribes often set apart or abandoned diseased members who were unable to contribute to communal social production. However, prior to the rise of the Judeo-Christian tradition, victims of disease were most often perceived as being personally guiltless. As sin and disease became associated, diseased individuals were increasingly seen as being guilty of religious or social deviancy, or social "otherness."

The association of disease and deviancy was reinforced by the discovery in the sixteenth century that venereal diseases were sexually transmitted. Henceforth, the treatment of individuals with venereal diseases mirrored societal attitudes toward sexual behavior.

During the Renaissance, a period of sexual tolerance, there was little stigma attached to one afflicted with a venereal disease. By the eighteenth century, however, with the rise of the middle class, and a corresponding emphasis on family values, a less tolerant attitude toward sex emerged. Sexually transmitted diseases were increasingly identified with "socially deviant behavior" (Dolan and Adams-Smith 1978).

Infectious epidemics predictably have resulted in demands for isolation of the individuals or groups affected, or perceived to be at risk or thought capable to transmitting the disease. They have traditionally unleashed pent-up social hatred toward individuals whose behavior is perceived to deviate from the dominant social norm. AIDS has followed this pattern. As Sontag notes: "Making AIDS everyone's problem and therefore a subject on which everyone needs to be educated . . . subverts our understanding of the difference between 'us' and 'them,' indeed exculpates or at least make irrelevant moral judgments about 'them' " (1988, 89).

Currently, discrimination against persons with AIDS (PWAs) and their families is based on the perception that "they" chose to have AIDS by participating in "deviant" behavior, that their behavior marks them as not "us" but "the other."[5]

The social mass created by discrimination acts to reinforce the constant creation of new categories of social "otherness." As discrimination spreads it is no longer linked to individual "deviancy" but is extended to entire "risk groups," gay and bisexual men, intravenous (I.V.) drug users, persons with hemophilia, and more recently women.

Social "otherness," related to AIDS, has transcended behavioral linkages. Blood product recipients and children (in spite of being seen as "innocent victims" of AIDS) are also labeled and treated as social "others."

Impoverished black and Latina women, who make up the majority of women diagnosed with AIDS, are not unfamiliar with being labeled "them" or "other." They experience such labeling repeatedly as immigrants, economically oppressed minorities, and members of cultures and subcultures whose traditional values hold them inferior or less economically and socially valued than males.

Historically, the creation of social "others," the stigmatization of the diseased, the racially despised, the economically disenfranchised, or the sexually feared, results in proposals for various forms of social control over their lives and behavior.[6]

Minority women in America's inner cities, already stigmatized by poverty, race, gender, and traditionally the targets of medical fertility control measures, understandably wish to avoid new forms of social control which are likely to accompany further stigmatization.

The need to avoid stigmatization takes the form of denial of risk, or it may result in adaptive behavior which mimics the dominant social norms, that is, the conferring of the label of social "otherness' on those in the community who engage in "deviant behavior" (an internalized form of victim-blaming).

In minority communities in New York City, those most often designated as "others" are gay and bisexual men, lesbians, and I.V. drug users. Black or Latina women who are lesbians and/or use I.V. drugs (and who may support their habits through prostitution) are especially labeled by "otherness."

## FEMALE I.V. DRUG USERS

Female I.V. drug users are perceived as being more "deviant" and are more negatively stereotyped than male I.V. drug users, even though they participate in a drug culture shaped by men who control the production and distribution of drugs. Traditionally, women have had less socioeconomic access to drugs and are most often introduced to needle use by men (Hser, Anglin, and McGlothlin 1987, 41).

Women I.V. users are not granted the same social status that male addicts receive for their risk-taking; they are punished more severely for their "social deviancy," and are considered harder to treat (Rosenbaum 1981a, 6–25).

Gender discrimination is common in drug treatment programs where the needs of female clients are not met by programs oriented to the needs of male I.V. users (Murphy and Rollins 1980, 320).[7] Treatment programs not only fail to address women's needs for female-oriented vocational training, child day care, assertiveness training, educational support and training, and health and social services (Burt, Glynn, and Sowder 1979), but they are hierarchical in nature, structured to require acceptance of an external locus of control. Female IVDUs with an internal locus of control are placed in opposition to the dominant (male) power structure of most treatment programs (Solomon 1982, 582).

In addition to being alienated from drug treatment, female I.V. users are often severed from natural support networks in their own communities. The criminalization of drug use makes it difficult for female I.V. users in minority communities, where there is limited access to employment and education opportunities, to participate productively in their own communities (Kail and Lukoff n.d., 6–8).[8]

Lesbian I.V. users in minority communities find themselves even more alienated, the ultimate social "others," stigmatized by religious approbation, conservative sexual mores, racism, sexism, and their lack of adherence to "traditional" gender roles. They are faced with choosing between repressing their sexual identity or losing their primary social support systems (Cornwell 1983, 106). The stigmatization of female I.V. drug users does not end when they stop using drugs, it follows them throughout their lives, turning them back to the drug world where they feel more comfortable (Biernacki 1986, 161).

The loss of social support systems by female I.V. users has serious implications as research indicates these networks play an important role in mediating in an I.V. drug-using career (Gerstein, Judd, and Rovner 1979).

Most research on female I.V. drug users, particularly that on minority women I.V. users, has been conducted from an orientation that equates drug use with social deviancy.[9]

There are alternative views of drug use that do not proceed from a deviancy model; drug use as a refuge from poverty, a correlate of domestic violence, a by-product of gender demands, or a means of economic survival.[10]

Drug use in minority communities is often viewed as a "competing life-style," an alternate economy, an adaptive response to poverty and racism (Tucker 1985, 1023).[11] This view is supported by Moore's study of Chicana female I.V. users on the West Coast, 77 percent of whom saw addiction as "just another way of life" (1988).[12]

This life-style takes its toll on female IVDUs. Heroin use weakens their self-esteem, leaving them open to maltreatment by male I.V. users (Cushey and Wathey 1982, 10). In females who use heroin, the drug tends to become the focal point of their relationships, undermining the relationships as sex-role boundaries are blurred and dissatisfaction with traditional gender-role behavior (which dictates "hysterical," sexual, helpless, or dependent behavior) grows (Solomon 1982, 582).[13]

Long-term heroin use itself has a negative effect on sexual functioning which contributes to women substituting heroin for sexual relations. Sexual dysfunction among female IVDUs is also related to sexual trauma—a significant number of female heroin addicts have experienced rape or incest prior to becoming addicts (Mondanaro et al. 1982, 312). Some researchers believe that I.V. use may be adopted as an escape from female sex-role expectations and sexual trauma, an escape into an asexual world (Singer 1974).

The research raises many questions about how gender-role expectations, and a community's response to them, impact on female IVDUs in different ethnic communities. Before examining these questions it is important to note that,

within ethnic groups, individual differences may be as salient as between-group cultural differences, and that within human collectives characterized as "black," "Latin" . . . etc. there may be significant variations in beliefs and behavior. (Bestman 1986, 217)

## LATINA WOMEN

There is a great deal of discussion of sex-role determinants among Latina women in the context of AIDS. However, most social science research on Latina sexuality has been problem-oriented, focusing on pregnancy and reproductive behavior, primarily among Mexican-Americans.[14]

This type of research does not express the fact that the United States has a broad spectrum of Latina women who belong to many distinct ethnic groups (and different social and economic classes within those groups), groups that do not necessarily interact with one another, which may in fact see one another as "others."

This, and the fact that there is a lack of research on sexual behavior and I.V. drug use among Latina women, means that there is limited material to draw on for an examination of the impact of cultural values on gender-role behavior as it relates to linkages between intravenous drug use, sexual behavior, and AIDS.

The present work focuses on what is known about Puerto Rican women in New York, where they make up the majority of Latina women who have been affected by AIDS. Puerto Rican women living in New York City share certain cultural experiences with other Latinas including:

1. The Spanish language;[15]

2. Spanish cultural domination, which transferred values that support gender roles championing male dominance (machismo);

3. Religion, in particular, Catholicism, which has had a strong impact on sexual mores (equating virginity with virtue), and which encourages fatalism (fatalismo);[16]

4. Immigration to the United States where they experience racism and economic oppression as minority members, and female members of a male-dominated society (Espin 1985, 153).

AIDS education in the Puerto Rican community has been hampered by the lack of insight by public health officials into how these experiences have affected sociocultural expectations and thus sexual and drug using behavior in the Puerto Rican community.

One of the first questions that needs to be explored is how traditional gender-role expectations have been affected by the educational and economic experiences of Puerto Rican women in New York City.

## Puerto Rican Gender Roles in New York City

Among Puerto Ricans living in New York City, culturally supported gender roles are based on traditional ideals which include an emphasis on the family and the gender-based concepts of *machismo* and *marianismo*.

*Machismo* involves an exaggerated sense of the importance of being male. This sense is instilled in male children at a very early age and is reinforced throughout the child's socialization. Boys are valued for simply being male and for assuming dominant roles in family dynamics and in their relationship with females (Medina 1987, 3).

Frequently, *machismo* has been mentioned as creating obstacles to the use of barrier methods of protection (condoms) by Latino males (Gross 1987, B5). Research indicates that many Puerto Rican males feel it is unmanly or unnatural to use such protection (Darabi 1986,12). Condom use is often perceived as unromantic; romance being culturally linked to impregnation and virility. The male proposing condom use may be seen as not "serious," that is, not desirous of pregnancy and marriage (Worth and Rodriquez 1987, 6).

*Marianismo* (the counterpart to *machismo*) "exalts chastity" and promotes girls being raised to be subservient, to cater to males (whether they be brothers, fathers, uncles, or husbands). Puerto Rican women are "constantly reminded of their inferiority and weakness and usually praised for their docility, submissiveness . . . and physical attractiveness" (Medina 1987, 3).

The ideal Puerto Rican woman centers her life on her husband and children, avoids sensuality, and is uncomfortable with sexual issues. Attractiveness and purity are synonymous. A Puerto Rican woman who is "prepared for sex" (e.g., carrying or asking for condoms to be used) may be perceived as undesirable or "loose" (ibid.).

Womanhood is traditionally equated with motherhood. It is through motherhood that the Puerto Rican woman can achieve social power, self-esteem, and community approval (Gatlin 1987, 184). Although some studies of young Puerto Rican women in New York City show that their concept of "womanhood" is changing, other studies indicate that this change is accompanied by high levels of stress (Canino 1982; Rosario 1982).

Counselors advising Puerto Rican women at high-risk for HIV infection to avoid or postpone pregnancy have to be aware of the possibly serious repercussions of such a suggestion, for both the women and their male partners (who may view impregnating a woman as proof of their virility [Arbona 1985, 9]).

The existence of a cultural double standard that emphasizes male sexuality and multiple female conquests while simultaneously disapproving of female enjoyment of sex creates a situation in which the male is less likely to respond to the desire of females to protect themselves against sexually transmitted diseases and pregnancy (ibid.).

The adherence to the traditional gender role among Puerto Rican women in New York varies widely. As early as the 1950s, sex-role behavior was undergoing changes in Puerto Rico itself. As U.S. influence increased, emphasis on the extended family diminished, and as female participation in the job market increased, traditional sex-role behavior came under pressure (Obeso and Bordatto 1979).

Sex-role behavior continues to be influenced by many factors including the degree of acculturation, access to economic and educational opportunities, the absence or presence of positive role models (the mother being an important role model), and the functional level of the family (McKenna and Ortiz 1988).

In high-conflict families, or families undergoing cultural or economic distress, females are more likely to act out and hold onto the nontraditional attitudes toward gender roles (Canino 1982, 17–31).[17]

### Latina I.V. Drug Users

Canino's research correlates with research on female Puerto Rican I.V. users, who were noted to be less concerned with their social desirability, less conforming to social roles, and more extroverted than their non-drug using counterparts (Messolonghites 1977).

This suggests that in addition to environmental factors (that is; large, disorganized, or single-headed families; drug use in the family; negative perceptions of the future based on the expectation of a lack of educational and economic opportunities; gender role stresses created by acculturation), Puerto Rican females who become involved in needle use may also be acting against traditional gender roles.[18]

To understand the female Puerto Rican I.V. user we have to look at the problems engendered by her acculturation to American culture, traditional cultural pressures in the Puerto Rican community, and her response to gender-role expectations.[19]

### Acculturation and Gender Roles

One of the primary changes that Latinas in the United States undergo comes about through their economic participation in the dominant culture. For Puerto

Rican women in New York City, this participation has been observed to decline as the number of female-headed households rises. Compared to other immigrants, Puerto Rican women have a lower rate of participation in the labor force. This has been attributed to the traditional family values which promote the role of mother and homemaker, but is more likely to be related to the low level of educational achievement among Puerto Rican females, their recent arrival in the United States, and economic declines in traditional forms of employment in New York City (Cooney and Colon 1980, 58–60).

McKenna and Ortiz (1988) explore the issue of Latina educational expectations and achievement, challenging many of the commonly held assumptions about the causes of lower levels of education achievement by Latinas. They find that structural barriers such as poor schooling play a dominant role in poor educational achievement. Their research indicated that Latinos' cultural beliefs support the desire for such achievement but that the awareness of the structural barriers result in a change in cultural expectations.

To understand changes in cultural expectations that have contributed to the creation of an increasing number of poor female-headed, single-parent families in the Puerto Rican community, it is necessary to examine the lessening of economic opportunities (a downturn in jobs in light manufacturing, the traditional sector of the economy in which Puerto Ricans in New York City are employed), and the precise causes of lower levels of educational achievement by Puerto Rican females (ibid., 38).[20]

Canino (1982) points to a disparity between professed cultural values and actual decision-making roles in the different Puerto Rican family systems she studied. She found more variation in *behavioral* values than in traditional *cultural* values. This has important implications for AIDS education, for it implies that while Puerto Ricans may express adherence to traditional cultural values such as *machismo* and *marianismo*, their behavioral choices may be based on other factors such as a decrease in male power related to unemployment.

The impact of structural barriers on cultural expectations and behavioral values varies among Latinos in New York City. Pessar (1986) has noted a different pattern of acculturation among Dominican women. Although the Dominican women she studied retained their traditional social roles as homemakers and mothers, they had the opportunity to expand these roles through employment outside the home. The lack of dichotomization between home and workplace worked to reduce gender tensions (such as those observed in the Puerto Rican community due to a lack of employment opportunities). The Dominican women in Pessar's study, as a result of their employment outside the home, shared more openly in family decision-making (Pessar 1986, 277, 296).

Castro's study of Colombian women living in New York City found their experience to be closer to that of Puerto Rican women. The economic opportunities open to them seem to have contributed to exacerbating intergenerational conflict, resulting in gender-role tensions. The Colombian men Castro studied were expected to make sexual decisions. The women are more socially segregated, their economic participation being downgraded to supplying what is seen as luxury items, objects not necessary for day-to-day survival. Castro saw the Colombian women she studied as being "objectified," providing objects, and who in turn objectify others, such as Puerto Ricans whom they consider socially inferior (Castro 1986, 242–49).

Although gender behavior is undergoing various levels of change related to economic and educational opportunities in different ethnic Latino communities in New York City, the cultural double standards created by the *machismo/ marianismo* roles continue to have some influence, particularly on sexual politics.

Sudden disruptions in these processes, through unemployment or addiction, can result in individual uncertainty, confusion, and conflict. The conflict is increased when an ethnic minority attempts to preserve their cultural uniqueness within the dominant majority.

The perceived threat to one's cultural uniqueness often results in a reinforcement of traditional cultural values, especially those related to sexual behavior. Stanton (1985) has observed that such values have changed slowly in the Puerto Rican community.[21]

## Puerto Rican Women and AIDS Education

Continued adherence to cultural, traditional gender roles, such as the prostitute/virgin dichotomy and the lack of social and economic value placed on females, which are reinforced by poverty and racism, contribute to placing Puerto Rican women at higher risk for the transmission of AIDS, especially in communities with high rates of I.V. drug use.

Ehrhardt has noted that men who perceive themselves as "macho" in any culture are more likely to be callous toward their sex partners, be involved in more sex-linked violence, have more partners, be more withdrawn emotionally, be less able to experience intimacy, be likely to pressure unwilling females into having sex relations, and have masturbation guilt (which is strongly correlated with refusal to use condoms) (Ehrhardt 1988). *Machismo* is also seen as a coverup for a low self-image: a form of overcompensating behavior and, when exaggerated, may be linked to drug use.

The continued existence of traditional sex-role dichotomies such as *machismo/ marianismo* indicates fears of unbridled sexual emotion which are reflected in the degree of homophobia observed among Latinos (Sundal-Hansen 1985, 217).[22]

Homosexuality is seen as chosen *bad behavior* such as drug use, a threat to the Puerto Rican male's sexual identity and the family's image. Homophobia is further reinforced by religious proscriptions on homosexuality. Although homosexual and bisexual behavior may be prevalent, homosexuality is still seen as being outside the cultural and religious norm.[23] Male dominance among Puerto Ricans and disdain for homosexuality are reinforced by Catholicism and fundamentalist Protestant religions. The Catholic Church, in particular, takes stances that promote homophobia and support the idea of a sexually subservient woman. The Virgin Mary (to feminists, a female symbol utilized by men to control women's sexual behavior) is proferred as a role model for Catholic women: the nonsexual, self-renunciating martyr-mother (Miles 1987, 4). We need to examine how structural changes are affecting gender-role behavior of individual women in Puerto Rican communities, and whether it is making it difficult for women to protect themselves against the sexual transmission of AIDS. Protection includes women discussing their sexual needs with partners, who may consider it out of character for women to discuss or exhibit an interest in sex.

Control of a woman's sexuality (*machismo* supports the perception that she is not able to control her own sexuality) is a family matter, with family honor tied to female purity and the oppression of female sexuality (Espin 1985).

When combined with economic powerlessness, racial discrimination, and physically dangerous environments, such cultural mores work together to support women's belief in their inability to control what happens to them. This belief is expressed and compounded by concepts such as *fatalismo*, a belief in fate or destiny (linked to the influence of Catholicism, but not limited to Latinos). *Espiritismo* must also be examined for the role it may play in helping to shape women's attitudes about personal control.

Impoverished Puerto Rican women, as minority members of the dominant culture, receive constant reinforcement for sex-role behavior which insinuates that they lack the power to directly affect or take control of their lives, or their sexuality, or to respond to aggression against them by oppressed frustrated males (Medina 1987,3).

Additionally, many Puerto Rican women are unable to correspond to the dominant culture's norm of beauty. This dilemma, when added to their social and economic disenfranchisement and the stigma that flows from a "victim-blaming" attitude prevalent in the 1980s, creates new forms of oppression that often become internalized as psychological oppression, affecting both ego strength and decision making.

The social stigma that accompanies AIDS threatens ego strength, self-image, and may be responded to fatalistically. It carries with it the threat of severance from traditional sociopsychological support systems, and the fear that disclosure of AIDS risk will bring "shame" on the entire family and the community.

The possibility of experiencing further "otherness" is personally threatening, and understandably can result in denial by Puerto Rican women at risk of the threat or reality of AIDS (Worth and Rodriquez 1987, 7).[24]

## BLACK WOMEN

A high degree of cultural variation exists between American, Haitian, other Caribbean, and African black women which needs to be explored in the context of AIDS prevention. This work limits itself to exploring the impact of dominant cultural values, racism, slavery, and a lack of opportunity for social and economic participation on the response of high-risk American black women to AIDS and AIDS education efforts.

In the United States, black females are often studied within the context of "social problems," and the women are presented as culturally inadequate and personally and socially disorganized (Hicks and Handler 1978, 315).[25]

The "history" of the relationship between blacks and diseases, as recorded by whites, is particularly instructive. The presence of syphilis among southern blacks was linked to their "immoral" behavior. The disease was linked to sexual behavior that could not or would not be controlled, therefore linked to individual character flaws (Hammonds 1987, 28).

The linkage of immorality and disease among blacks was not limited to sexually transmitted diseases. In nineteenth-century Virginia, the spread of cholera was connected with the ". . . supposed degraded condition, sinful ways, and filthy habits" of free blacks and slaves, who were considered ". . . deserving of such a plague" by white Virginians who related ". . . high morals, clean living, and religious orthodoxy" to their own supposed "immunity" to the disease (Savitt 1978, 227). These attitudes extended to perceptions of the "educatability" of blacks concerning health.

Officials, newspaper editors, and charitable groups felt that despite their attempts to teach blacks proper precautions and treatments, these people remained impudent. They refused to change their habits in the face of impending danger, much to the detriment of themselves, their masters, and the public. (ibid., 231)

Researchers and historians continue to have difficulty in distinguishing cultural and religious variables from the structural variables that affect black women's choices (Jones 1985, 173). Although economic and social survival exert strong influences on both sexual and risk-taking behavior in the black community, there has been little exploration of the social or economic determinants of attitudes toward sex and drug use among black women (Fox-Genovese 1988). Too often, the behavior of black women is filtered through cultural stereotypes.

## Community Responses to Sexual Stereotyping

One response in the black community to social and racial stereotypes has been the avoidance of open discussion of sexual behavior and drug use. Homosexuality and bisexuality are dealt with in "a very conservative . . . fashion" (Hammonds 1987, 31).[26] This has important implications for AIDS education. Bakeman et al. note that blacks, like other people of color, would rather report that they are IV drug users than gay. Furthermore, they have reported that 30 percent of their black male patients with AIDS were bisexual (Houston-Hamilton 1986, 2). Hammonds has suggested that bisexual men have the highest number of sexual encounters in the black community (ibid.).

Black homosexuals, bisexuals, and drug users are often designated "others" within their own community, which has internalized the stigma it experiences in dominant American culture. As in the Latino and white communities, negative attitudes toward homosexuality are reinforced by religious beliefs that view homosexuality and drug use as deviant or sinful behavior.

The stigma of homosexuals and IVDUs, as Hammonds notes, affects the entire black community as it leads to AIDS being perceived as another example of "bad behavior" or "otherness," a subject not to be openly discussed.

Silence surrounding homosexuality and drug use in the black community poses a real challenge to AIDS prevention. It affects efforts for behavior modification such as condom ("rubber") use which may be equated with homosexuality or an implement of genocide (in the tradition of the forced sterilization of black women).

## Black Women, Gender, Race, and Culture

The cultural values that inform sexuality among American black women cannot be understood out of the context of racism, sexism, and economic oppression which have shaped black gender relations and family structure.

The impact of slavery, the exploitation of the productive and reproductive rights of black females, the vulnerability of black communities in attempting to protect their traditional gender relations, the impact of illiteracy and lack of access to education, differing northern and southern social experiences, and the changes in family structure resulting from northern migration after World War II have all played a role in shaping gender relations and family structure (Fox-Genovese 1988, 373).[27] Only recently, as historians have explored women's history, is the influence of these and other events on black female gender-role behavior being explored and debated. Researchers are handicapped in this endeavor, however, by the "sparse and often biased sources" (Woodward 1988, 3).

The research that has emerged indicates that black gender politics have been affected by black women being "alienated from and bound to the dominate white model of womanhood . . . ," the internalization of sexual stereotypes applied by whites, paternalistic domination—resulting in devaluation of the female body (and exploitation and abuse of black women), and the "colonization" of values concerning appearance (such as seeing lighter women with straight hair as being more sexually desirable) (Fox-Genovese 1988, 194; Houston-Hamilton 1988; Williams 1985, 104–6).

Over the last hundred years blacks have been subjected to various stereotypes, including the myth of hypersexuality. One response to such stereotyping, and to the exploitation of black women by white men, has been the adoption of conservative sexual mores by some black women.

The myth of black women's sexuality is turned back upon them in the form of sexual prudery, with black women becoming alienated from both their own bodies and sexual desires (Spillers 1985, 76).[28] Alienation is exacerbated by socialization patterns in the black community which encourage women to subordinate their needs and desires to those of men. Gatlin and others promote the idea that the most important aspect of a black woman's life is often perceived to be "her relationship with a man" (Gatlin 1987, 138, 179).[29]

Dependence on male validation, (the feeling that life is meaningless without a man) when combined with a black male's sense of rage at his powerlessness in the face of racism and economic disenfranchisement, can lead to abuse; that abuse becomes a "substitute" for long-term monogamous relationships (Gordon 1985, 18).

The dependence on male validation can be complicated by a shortage of males in many black communities. Black women, where such a shortage exists, may have discontinuous sexual relations (i.e., they may have to share men).[30] The discontinuity of opportunities for intimate (sexual) contact means such opportunities are highly valued, making it hard to insist on female desires such as the use of barrier protection (i.e., condoms) if one has a resistant partner. A shortage of males can mean that "many black women have to take love on male terms," a situation that supports sexual exploitation of black women (Hine and Wittenstein 1981, 344).

## Black Women and Religion

Black churches serve as a foundation for the community's value system (especially as it relates to survival), helping to maintain group unity and foster self-respect in the face of continuing racism. Because black churches are agents for social control and socialization, their participation in addressing the problem of AIDS in the black community is crucial (Allen et al. 1981, 90).

Religion plays a major supporting role in many black women's sexual behavior. Jackson et al. note that as many as 80 percent of black women use prayer as a primary resource to cope with personal problems. Black women draw emotional strength from participation in diverse churches which have played a major role in their socialization. Churches offer women the opportunity to express themselves, to be recognized; they act as women's primary source of social support, and help women gain self-esteem through self-help.

Furthermore, research indicates that religion is an important variable in nondrug use by black females (Rosenberg, Karl, and Berberian 1974, 73–96). This was confirmed by IV drug users who were interviewed by the author about the resources that exist to help adolescents not to become involved in drug use in communities where drugs are pervasive.

Religion also influences gender behavior through sexism experienced in church participation, and through the influence of the Bible, which is often used as the basis for determining religiously "correct" behavior (some believe that it promotes the idea of male dominance and considers non-procreative sexual behavior sinful). Furthermore, individual churches can act in a manner

that reinforces sexual conservatism (becoming a substitute for personal interactions that are too socially or sexually threatening) (Gordon 1985, 17).[31]

## Black Female IVDUs

Intravenous drug use among black women, like that among Latina women,
has been studied from a perspective of deviant behavior. Most of the research
has been conducted in drug treatment or prison programs resulting in the study
of black female IVDUs disembodied from their natural environments.[32]

There is insufficient research on the variation that exists in drug use between
different groups of black women, the effect of cocaine succeeding heroin as a
drug of choice of black women IVDUs, or the cultural, religious or economic
variables which influence female drug use (Kail and Lukoff n.d., 9).[33]

Predictors of IV drug use among black women are said to include: dropping
out of school, marijuana use at a young age, a history of delinquency, dealing
drugs, coming from a broken home, and having an IVDU in the family (Chambers and Harter 1987, 207–8). These predictors are symptoms of poverty and
lack of access to economic and educational opportunities, a lack of cultural
expectations that things can be different.

A study of black women IVDUs by Moise, Kovach, Reed, and Bellows (1982),
found that heroin injection was more likely to be the result of *economic* and
*social deprivation* among black females. They also have more access to injectable
drugs. Moise et al., found black women IV drug users tend to use heroin the
first time using a drug as they are able to buy heroin on the street.

## Addiction and Gender-Role Behavior

The relationship between gender-role expectations and drug use among black
female IVDUs is unclear. One study of black female IVDUs found that female
heads of households tend to follow "traditional gender-role expectations," mar-
rying prior to becoming addicted. The adherence to "traditional gender-role
expectations" was also true of female IVDUs who pursued conventional life-
styles. A third group, who chose the "fast life," did not follow traditional gender
behavior. Their behavior was similar to IV-using males involved in crime. The
behavior of the third group is most likely to be studied, or taken for the norm,
as these women have the most contact with institutions involved in addressing
"social deviancy" (Kail and Lukoff n.d., 8).

Chambers, Dean, and Pletcher's study of black female heroin addicts indicated
that their criminal behavior differed from that of black male heroin addicts,
although the same proportion of men and women IVDUs were involved in
committing property crimes. The women were more focused in the type of
crimes they committed, less "opportunistic," and less assaultive. Both sexes were
heavily involved in drug dealing (1987, 465). The most frequently committed
crime by black IVDUs was prostitution (ibid., 466). The younger women were

more likely to commit crimes against persons, the older women more likely to be dealing drugs (ibid., 470).[34]

Kail and Lukoff's study indicates there is variation in gender behavior among addicts. The subject should be further researched and linked to exploring the social or economic impact of being unmarried, single, or unemployed in the black community, and its possible role in leaving black women more vulnerable to addiction (Jackson, Neighbors, and Gurin 1986, 100). Fillilove (1988) and Andriote (1988) note that it is often culturally unacceptable for a black woman (Haitian-American in the case of Andriote) not to have a male partner, that the perceived need for a partner is paramount. We need to understand the relationship between that perceived need and survival in inner city communities with illicit economies that are male-dominated. Is having a male partner an important component of a woman's survival strategy in these communities?

## AIDS Education and Black Women

AIDS education that promotes "safer sex" may threaten behavior patterns that black women link with their survival. The suggestion that black women should explore new forms of sexual behavior as a means of prevention of HIV transmission may be received ambivalently by women subject to victim-blaming because of stereotypes about their "supposed" sexual behavior. Victim-blaming and sexual exploitation have resulted in some black women choosing abstinence or chastity (Hine and Wittenstein 1981, 289).

Currently, there is insufficient knowledge about patterns of sexual behavior among poor black women in our inner cities; the information that does exist is often contradictory. Houston-Hamilton (1988) has observed that poor black women may have more limited sexual repertoires than white women. They may equate intimacy specifically with vaginal sex or penetration. An emphasis on vaginal sex relates to an orientation to procreation rather than erotic sex, an orientation supported by conservative religious values. It is an important observation, one that needs to be explored.

## Social Distrust and AIDS Prevention in the Black Community

AIDS prevention efforts in the black community must not only be based on an understanding of the effect of poverty, racism, and economic oppression on sexual decision-making and role behavior, such efforts must also overcome the low level of trust in health care professionals and health services.

Distrust of public health services in the black community has a long history. From the time that blacks were brought to the United States as slaves, parallel black and white medical beliefs and practices existed. Their traditional medical practices were first employed by blacks on plantations in the South so as not to let the white masters know they were ill. These practices were often less invasive than many official or "white" medical practices that were actually damaging to their health.

Today, distrust of health services by black women is related to the belief in the black community that—should an individual discuss their "business" with whites—whites will use what is told them to hurt or blame the black individual. This belief reflects the experience of black Americans that unless a health problem affects the white community it is seldom addressed in the black community.

The response of black women to personal risk for AIDS must be considered in the context of the risks associated with living with sexism, racism, and socioeconomic oppression on a daily basis, of constantly being reminded that one is distinct from and "inferior" to the majority, and that one has limited access to addressing one's needs. Black women's wariness of self-disclosure is part of their larger survival strategy. AIDS must address that survival strategy in order to break down denial which is driven by fear of racial and sexual backlash if women admit to being at risk.

Denial does not just exist on an individual level, it is cumulative. Unless the community in which black women live can afford to face the impact of AIDS, free from further discrimination, free from the fear that by addressing the problem of AIDS the black community will open itself to furthering the traditional association of blacks, disease, and "immoral behavior," denial of the risk of AIDS and the ensuing conspiracy of silence about it will continue. Who delivers the message that AIDS is an issue of importance to the black community, and that institution's or individual's political beliefs about the etiology of AIDS, will determine how or whether that message is received and acted upon.

## CROSS-CULTURAL COMMONALITIES RELATED TO AIDS PREVENTION

In order for AIDS education to be effective it has to be based on an understanding of the relationship between individuals and their social worlds. Ignoring these relationships contributes to creating barriers to women participating fully in AIDS prevention (Tesh 1988).

Other barriers are created by outdated paradigms of disease etiology. For instance, implicit in the idea that AIDS or other diseases are the result of "bad personal behavior," such as IV drug use, is the assumption that the government or society cannot address the roots of IV drug use in poverty, racism, and sexism.

By accepting this paradigmatic view of disease causation, individuals and communities may unwittingly contribute to the depolitization of AIDS transmission. Such a viewpoint assumes that individuals, even impoverished minority groups members, have adequate resources to lead a healthy life and to engage in personal AIDS risk reduction (Tesh 1988, 24).[35] It ignores the evidence that the vast changes in the ability to deal with infectious disease have resulted in improvements in the standard of living (the removal of structural barriers to good health).

Impoverished black and Latina women live in unpredictable environments which are physically and emotionally threatening. Distrust of extra-familial, community resources or programs may be part of a woman's survival strategy. Women's distrust of public health services and education reflect the feeling that they have been denied access to sufficient power to control their environment, that seeking help will "embarrass" them or their family, that their efforts are not likely to bring about the results they desire.

Distrust contributes to a delay in women seeking services, a lack of planning for health care and other social needs, an orientation toward the present, and beliefs that there are proper ways of behavior which produce the desired results.[36] Perceiving a lack of flexibility or choices can promote fatalism.[37]

AIDS educators who do not offer programs building on the strengths of black and Latina women, who do not offer choices and cultural flexibility, place the women they are trying to engage in behavior change in the position of making often untenable choices (e.g., get your partner to wear a condom—or get AIDS). Black and Latina women not only need to be offered help to reconcile their traditional cultural roles with their needs to learn how to talk with partners about how to protect themselves from AIDS, and if they are not able to convince a partner to wear a condom, to minimize their risk through other actions.

Women need help in addressing the impact of IV drug use on their families and communities. Promoting condom use as the main thrust of AIDS prevention is not good enough. It ignores that the vast majority of educated white American women do not or cannot get their partners to wear condoms, and it ignores the links between class and disease prevention in the United States. AIDS education has to offer women living in communities with large numbers of HIV-infected males culturally appropriate role models and combine the use of role models with programs which address the real need for health care, education, and job opportunities to which many women have no access.

AIDS educators must keep in mind that sexual choices express not only cultural values and expectations but adaptive means of living with racism, sexism, and economic disenfranchisement. Introducing behavioral concepts that propose to alter or go against cultural values or ignore structural variables can lead to social conflict, especially in communities undergoing rapid acculturation.[38]

Proposed changes in gender roles or sexual behavior may create guilt over acting against traditional community norms and set in motion changes that will alter the locus of power in sexual relationships. The sex lives of many minority women are currently characterized by a lack of power, by multiple forms of "otherness" that are imposed on them from within and without their community. If they are to be supported to undertake behavior changes, their "otherness" has to be diminished, and behavior changes must be linked to the attitudes and beliefs that support their concepts of cultural and economic survival.

AIDS education targeted at minority women, if it is not based on the knowledge of cultural values and gender politics, will further increase high-risk behavior if individual women feel that their economic and social survival mechanisms are threatened by acknowledging risk-related behavior that they feel powerless to alter. It is not sufficient to study cultural and gender roles and beliefs as they affect women. A methodological approach is needed to enable us to look at the socialization of both females and males and its collective impact on sexual behavior.

The effect of acculturation and racism on family structure and gender-role expectations in different ethnic groups has to be examined further. Only when the knowledge generated by such research is available will public health educators be able to fully understand how different individuals make decisions about behavior based on communal norms that determine their response to AIDS and AIDS education.

## NOTES

1. Anthropologists can contribute to AIDS prevention program development by helping to interpret how social interaction and behavior are influenced by poverty and racism, and how responses to both vary across cultures. They can examine shared values, rules and behavioral expectations, and help program developers to understand the cultural values and traditions which legitimize behavior choices related to AIDS.

2. Cross-cultural research on cultural beliefs and attitudes toward illness, disease, and health care as they relate to AIDS service provision is also important but cannot be addressed in the present inquiry.

3. Eighty-five percent of female AIDS deaths in New York City are Latina and black, the majority of Latinas being Puerto Rican and the majority of blacks are U.S.-born.

Puerto Ricans born in Puerto Rico make up 52 percent of all Latino AIDS deaths in New York City. Health Department data are not broken down so that U.S.-born Puerto Rican AIDS deaths can be separated from those of other Latinos. Estimates are that of the remaining 48 percent, approximately 24 percent are U.S.-born Puerto Ricans. This means that Puerto Ricans in New York City make up 76 percent of all Latino AIDS deaths.

4. Since 1986, the author has been engaged in research on the barriers to AIDS-related behavior change among high-risk women in several programs; one run in conjunction with the New York City Department of Health at the Stuyvesant Polyclinic in Lower Manhattan, one for women heroin addicts in methadone maintenance at Montefiore Medical Center in the Bronx, and an outreach project, sponsored by Narcotic and Drug Research, Inc., which worked with intravenous drug using women and prostitutes on Manhattan's Lower East Side. The programs promote AIDS risk reduction in high-risk women through participation in peer-based groups focused on social skill building and street outreach.

5. This viewpoint led to the burden of addressing AIDS prevention falling on those perceived to be most at risk, originally gay men. More recently, it is obscuring the need to address the social factors that promote drug use in the inner city neighborhoods.

6. As is also true today, throughout history, female prostitutes have often been one

of the first targets of social control. During the sixteenth century, for instance, they were expelled from towns. In seventeenth-century Brazil when a yellow fever epidemic occurred, prostitutes were jailed or exiled while other women were confined to their homes (Tesh 1988, 13). More recently, prostitutes were incarcerated during World War I.

7. Only about 20 percent of I.V. drug using women enter drug treatment (Cushey and Wathey 1982, 4).

For a discussion of the special needs of I.V. drug using women entering treatment, see: Beschner, G. M., Reed, B. G., and Mondanaro, J., eds., *Treatment Services for Drug Dependent Women*, Vol. I, NIDA, DHHS, Washington, 1981 and Reed, B. G., Beschner, G. M., and Mondanaro, J., eds., *Treatment Services for Drug Dependent Women*, Vol. II, NIDA, DHHS, Washington, 1982.

8. Escamilla-Mondanaro, in speaking about the socialization of female heroin addicts notes that they suffer from "strict sex-role socialization" reinforced by social oppression, sexism, racism, and classism which give them negative messages about self-esteem, foster alienation, dependency, and lack of self-confidence (1977).

9. There are multiple drug abuse paradigms; biochemical, psychological, sociological, socio-psychological, and symbolic. See Biernacki (1986, 12–36).

10. Research such as that conducted by Cushey and Wathey (1982, 11) on female I.V. users portrays them as typically the partners of male I.V. users, exhibiting a greater degree of dependence, being less assertive, and suffering more from depression than the male users. This view is contradicted by other research; see Chabon (1987).

11. Research indicates that environmental influences on drug use are greater in minority communities than in white communities (Tucker 1985, 1033).

12. Moore notes that another 19 percent of women interviewed had found I.V. users "exciting" role figures when they were younger (1988, 9).

13. Rosenbaum has noted the ability of heroin-using women to earn more money through prostitution than their male partners as one factor in the disruption of sex-role behavior (1981b, 1197–1206).

14. Existing research portrays Chicana women as less knowledgeable about sex and contraception, less likely to receive sexual information in the family and to talk with their partners about sex, and more likely to desire a greater number of children than their Anglo counterparts (Amaro 1988).

15. Espin makes a salient observation on the importance of language in working with Puerto Rican women on issues that require discussing intimate behavior. She notes that although conversing in a second language about intimacy may be uncomfortable, it may be easier for women to discuss explicit sexual behavior that is too threatening to discuss in one's primary language (Espin 1985, 152–53).

16. Approximately 85 percent of Latinos are nominally Catholic (Medina 1987, 1). In New York, however, a growing number of evangelical churches have attracted Puerto Ricans. See, Stevens-Arroyo, A. M., "Puerto Rican Struggles in the Catholic Church," *The Puerto Rican Struggle*, Rodriquez et al., eds., 1980.

17. Family function also influences how the threat of AIDS is responded to. Dysfunctional families may adaptively employ denial as a means of helping the family member with AIDS without having to confront the behavior that put the member at risk for the disease.

18. Zahn and Ball (1974, 211–12) on the other hand note that I.V. drug use is not necessarily linked with "deviant" gender behavior among Puerto Rican women, some of whom continue to conform to role expectations.

19. Ten years ago Bullington observed that sex-role dependency among Chicanas carried over into drug use; female addicts depended on men to get them their drugs and to inject them. This had implications for relationships as their cessation meant a disruption in the women's drug use (1977, 85). There is a need to update such work and provide cross-cultural comparisons between different ethnic groups of Latina women.

20. If the male does not fulfill expectations as a provider or family head, a Puerto Rican woman can and does ask him to leave, and will support herself and family—on welfare if necessary.

21. Bestman (1986) notes that Puerto Ricans are generally of lower socioeconomic origins, more racially mixed, residentially segregated, and "more rigidly cast in traditional family relationships" than Cubans in Miami (p. 207).

22. The degree of homophobia varies among Latinos. In the Puerto Rican community in New York City, it is very high.

23. Forty-seven percent of Latino males with AIDS in New York City are listed as having had sex with a man at risk (New York City Department of Health AIDS Surveillance, March 30, 1988).

24. Denial is not an exclusive response of any particular group threatened by AIDS; it "has characterized the response of every group" (Goldstein 1987, 19).

25. It is beyond the scope of the present work to examine the cross-cultural difference between American, Haitian, and Caribbean blacks.

26. This conservatism is also found among black feminists who have sometimes acted as spokeswomen for "prudery" as respectability to counteract the sexual exploitation of black women by both black and white men (DuBois and Gordon 1985, 41).

27. This did not stop black males from attempting to protect black females from white owners or from suffering the consequences (Fox-Genovese 1988, 49).

28. These experiences have also created alternative behavior models. Oppression resulted in black men and women having to work together to survive. Communal life has acted as a transforming agent for some black women, who help one another become "moral agents who help to redefine values from the perspective of their own experience" (Williams 1985, 92).

29. The belief that a man is the most important thing in a woman's life is not limited to black women. Social commentators continually stress that relationships are more important to American women while work is more important to men.

30. The shortage is related to the high number of black men who are killed, or are imprisoned. See Hacker (1988) for a discussion of this issue.

31. Unlike the Catholic Church in Latino communities, there is no one monolithic church structure in the black community which is a culturally pervasive influence. Black churches speak in many voices (Fillilove, 1988).

32. This research, much of it conducted before 1966, when the treatment of addicts shifted from the federal government to the states, indicated that for their proportion in the population blacks were "over-represented" among IVDUs, and that intravenous drug use was concentrated in New York and New Jersey (Chambers et al. 1987, 195).

33. The use of cocaine has increased 50 percent since 1975 and is correlated to an increasing amount of crime committed by female IVDUs (Sanchez and Johnson 1986, 14).

34. Chambers, Dean, and Pletcher found the same pattern in Chicana IVDUs (1987, 477).

35. This approach also echoes the American belief in individual autonomy.

36. There is a perceived difference in the time orientation of minorities. Blacks are perceived to be more present oriented than the Chinese who are perceived as being past/future oriented.

37. A study of adolescents found Puerto Rican adolescents had the most rigid behavior norms of three groups studied (whites, blacks, and Puerto Ricans). This could be related to stronger adherence to traditional concepts of gender-linked behavior (Messolonghites 1977, 16).

38. The faster acculturation of Latino children is noted as playing a role in drug use, as traditional family values are upset, leaving adolescents more vulnerable to peer pressure (Tucker 1985, 1034).

## REFERENCES

Allen, Marie L., et al. 1981. "Perceptions of Problematic Behavior by Southern Female Black Fundamentalists and Mental Health Professionals," In *Biocultural Aspects of Disease*, Rothschild, H. ed. New York: Academic Press, pp. 87–90.

Amaro, Hortensia. 1988. "Implications of Sexual and Contraceptive Practices/Attitudes for Prevention of Heterosexual Transmission in Hispanics," NIDA Technical Review Meeting on Heterosexual Spread of HIV Infection and AIDS in the United States, January 19–20.

Andriote, John-Manuel. 1988. "For Women At Risk, Prevention Begins With Self-Esteem," *The NAN Monitor*, vol. 3 (1), Fall, Washington, D.C., p. 15.

Anglin, M. Douglas, Hser, Yih-Ing, and McGlothlin, William 1987. "Sex Differences in Addict Careers. 2. Becoming addicted," *American Journal of Drug and Alcohol Abuse*, vol. 13 (1 & 2), pp. 59–71.

Arbona, Rebecca. 1985. "Adolescent Pregnancy: An Overview," Hispanic Women's Center, August, pp. 1–10.

Bestman, Evalina, W. 1986. "Cross-Cultural Approaches to Service Delivery to Ethnic Minorities: The Miami Model," In *Mental Health Research and Practice in Minority Communities*, Miranda, M. R., and Kitano, H. H., eds. DHHS, National Institute of Mental Health, Rockville, pp. 199–226.

Biernacki, Patrick. 1986. *Pathways From Heroin Addiction Recovery Without Treatment.* Temple University Press, Philadelphia, pp. 12–161.

Bullington, Bruce. 1977. *Heroin Use in the Barrio.* Lexington Books, Lexington, MA, p. 85.

Burt, M. R., Glynn, T. J., and Sowder, B. J. 1979. "Psychosocial Characteristics of Drug-Abusing Women," NIDA, DHEW, Washington, D.C.

Canino, Glorisa. 1982. "Transactional Family Patterns: A Preliminary Exploration of Puerto Rican Female Adolescents," In *Work, Family and Health: Latina Women in Transition*, Zambrana, R. ed. Hispanic Research Center, Fordham University, Monograph No. 7., pp. 27–36.

Castro, Mary G. 1986. "Work versus Life: Colombian Women in New York," In *Women and Change In Latin America*, Nash, J., and Safa, H. eds. Bergin and Garvey Publishers, South Hadley, pp. 242–49.

Chabon, Brenda. 1987. "Cognitive Distortions in Depressed and Suicidal Drug Abusers." *International Journal of the Addictions*, vol. 21 (12), pp. 1313–29.

Chambers, Carl D., Dean, Sara W., and Pletcher, Michael F. 1987. "Criminal Involvements of Minority Group Addicts," in *Chemical Dependencies*, pp. 464–83.

Chambers, Carl D., and Harter, Michael T. 1987. "The Epidemiology of Narcotic Abuse Among Blacks in the United States 1935–1980," in *Chemical Dependencies*, Chambers, Carl D., et al., eds., Ohio University Press, Athens, pp. 191–208.

Chambers, Carl D., Hinesley, R. K., and Moledestad, Mary. 1970. "Narcotic Addiction In Females: A Race Comparison," *International Journal of the Addictions*, vol. 5, (2), pp. 257–75, June.

Cooney, Rosemary S., and Colon, Alice. 1980. "Work and Family: The Recent Struggle of Puerto Rican Females," In *The Puerto Rican Struggle: Essays on Survival in the U.S.*, Rodriquez, C. E., Korrol, V. S., and Alers, J. O., eds. Maplewood, N.J.: Waterfront Press. pp. 53–73.

Cornwell, Anita. 1983. *Black Lesbian in White America*. Tallahassee, FL; The NAIAD Press, p. 106.

Cushey, Walter R., and Wathey, Richard B. 1982. *Female Addiction*. Lexington Books, Lexington, P. 5.

Darabi, Katherine F. 1986. "Strategies For Improving Access To Family Planning Services: A Case Study of Service Barriers for Hispanic Youth," Governor's Conference on the Multi-Cultural Family of New York, Albany, June 19.

Dolan, John P., and Adams-Smith, William N. 1978. *Health and Society: A Documentary History of Medicine*. The Seabury Press, New York.

DuBois, Ellen C., and Gordon, Linda. 1985. "Seeking Ecstasy on the Battlefield: Danger and Pleasure in Nineteenth Century Feminist Sexual Thought," In *Pleasure and Danger*, Vance C., ed. Routledge and Kegan Paul, Boston, p. 31.

Ehrhardt, Anke. 1988. "Implications of Sexual and Contraceptive Practices/Attitudes For Prevention of Heterosexual Transmission in Men in Heterosexual Relationships," NIDA Technical Review Meeting, January 29–20.

Eldred, C. A., and Washington, M. N. 1975. "Female Heroin Addicts in a City Treatment Program: The Forgotten Minority." *Psychiatry*, vol. 38 (1) pp. 75–85.

Escamilla-Mondanaro, J. 1977. "Women: Pregnancy, Children and Addiction," *Journal of Psychedelic Drugs*, vol. 9 (1), pp. 55–68.

Espin, Olivia M. 1985. "Cultural and Historical Influences on Sexuality in Hispanic/Latin Women: Implications for Psychotherapy," In *Pleasure and Danger*, Vance, C., ed. Routledge and Kegan Paul, Boston, pp. 149–64.

Fillilove, Mindy. 1988. Personal communication, November.

Fox-Genovese, Elizabeth. 1988. *Within The Plantation Household*. University of North Carolina Press, Chapel Hill, pp. 39–53.

Gatlin, Rochelle. 1987. *American Women Since 1945*. University of Mississippi Press, Jackson, pp. 138–84.

Gerstein, D. R., Judd, L. L., and Rovner, S. A. 1979. "Career Dynamics of Female Heroin Addicts," *American Journal of Drug and Alcohol Abuse*, vol. 6 (1), pp. 1–23.

Goldstein, Richard. 1987. "AIDS and Race," *The Village Voice*, March 10, p. 19.

Gordon, Vivian V. 1985. *Black Women, Feminism and Black Liberation: Which Way?* Third World Press, Chicago, pp. 17–68.

Griffin-Shelly, Eric, 1986. "Sex Roles in Addiction: Defense or Deficit," *International Journal of the Addictions*, vol. 21 (2), pp. 1307–12.

Gross, Jane. 1987. "Bleak Lives: Women Carrying AIDS," *New York Times*, August 27, pp. A1, B5.

Hacker, Andrew. 1988. "Black Crime, White Racism," *New York Review of Books*, vol. 35 (3), March 3, pp. 36–41.

Hammonds, Evelyn. 1987. "Race, Sex, AIDS: The Construction of Other," *Radical America*, vol. 20 (6), November, pp. 28–36.

Hicks, George L., and Handler, Mark J. 1978. "Ethnicity, Public Policy, and Anthropologists," In *Applied Anthropology in America*, Eddy, E., and Partridge W. eds. Columbia University Press, New York, pp. 292–312.

Hine, Darlene, and Wittenstein, Kate. 1981. "Female Slave Resistance: The Economics of Sex," In *The Black Women Cross-Culturally*, Steady, Filomina, ed. Schenkman Publishing Company, Cambridge, 289–344.

Houston-Hamilton, Amanda, 1988. "Implications of Sexual and Contraceptive Practices/Attitudes for Prevention of Heterosexual Transmission in Blacks," NIDA Technical Review Meeting, January 19–20.

———. 1986. "A Constant Increase: AIDS In Ethnic Communities," Focus, vol. 1 (11), October, pp. 1–2.

Hser, Yih-Ing, Anglin, M. Douglas, and McGlothlin, William. 1987. "Sex Differences in Addict Careers. 1. Initiation of Use," *American Journal of Drug and Alcohol Abuse*, vol. 13 (1 & 2), pp. 33–57.

Jackson, James S., Neighbors, Harold W., and Gurin, Gerald. 1986. "Findings From A National Survey of Black Mental Health: Implications for Practice and Training," in *Mental Health Research in Minority Communities*, Miranda, M. R., and Kitano, H. H., eds. National Institute of Mental Health, Rockville, pp. 91–116.

Jones, Enrico E. 1985. "Psychotherapy and Counseling with Black Clients," In *Handbook of Cross-Cultural Counseling and Therapy*, Pederson, P., ed. Praeger, New York, p. 173.

Kail, Barbara L., and Lukoff, Irving F. n.d. "The Female Addict's Career Options: A Typology and Theory," Narcotic and Drug Research, New York Division of Substance Abuse, pp. 1–9.

Lorde, Audre. 1984. *Sister Outsider*. The Crossing Press, Trumansburg, pp. 48–60.

McKenna, Teresa, and Ortiz, Flora, eds. 1988. *The Broken Web: The Educational Experience of Hispanic American Women*. Berkeley, CA: The Tomas Rivera Center and Floricanto Press.

Medina, Carmen. 1987. "Latino Culture and Sex Education," SIECUS Report, January-February, vol. 15 (3), pp. 1–3.

Messolonghites, Louisa. 1977. *Multicultural Perspectives on Drug Abuse and Its Prevention: A Resource Book*. NIDA DHEW, Washington, pp. 8–16.

Miles, Margaret R. 1987. "Introduction." *Immaculate and Powerful*, Atkinson, C. W., Buchanan, C. H., and Miles, M. R., eds. Beacon Press, Boston, pp. 3–5.

Moise, R., Kovad, R. J., Reed, B. G., and Bellows, N. 1982. "A Comparison of Black and White Women Entering Drug Abuse Treatment Programs." *The International Journal of Addictions*, vol. 7 (1), pp. 35–49.

Mondanaro et al. 1982. "Sexuality and Fear of Intimacy as Barriers to Recovery for Drug Dependent Women." In *Treatment Services for Drug Dependent Women*, vol. 2, DHHS, NIDA, Washington, D.C., pp. 312–13.

Moore, Joan. 1988. "Chicana Addicts." Unpublished manuscript, Sociology Department, University of Wisconsin, Milwaukee.

Murphy, Leonard, and Rollins, Joan H. 1980. "Attitudes Toward Women In Co-Ed and

All Female Drug Treatment Programs," *Journal of Drug Education*, vol. 10 (4), p. 320.

Obeso, P., and Borelatta, D. 1979. "Cultural Implications in Treating the Puerto Rican Female." *American Journal of Drug and Alcohol Abuse*, vol. 6 (3), pp. 337–44.

Pessar, Patricia, 1986. "The Role of Gender in Dominican Settlement in the United States." In *Women and Change in Latin America*, Nash, J., and Safa, H. eds. Bergin and Garvey Publishers, South Hadley, pp. 276–77.

Rosario, L. M. 1982. "The Self-Perception of Puerto Rican Women Toward Their Societal Roles." In *Work, Family and Health: Latina Women in Transition*, Zambrana, R. E., ed. Hispanic Research Center, Fordham University, pp. 11–16.

Rosenbaum, Marsha. 1981a. *Women On Heroin*. Rutgers University Press, Rutgers, pp. 6–25.

————. 1981b. "When Drugs Come into the Picture, Love Flies out the Window; Women Addicts' Love Relationships." *International Journal of the Addictions*, vol. 16 (7) pp. 1197–1206.

Rosenberg, Janis, Karl, Stanislav V., and Berberian, Roslie M. 1974. "Sex Differences in Adolescent Drug Use: Recent Trends," *Addictive Diseases: An International Journal*, vol. 1 (10), pp. 73–96.

Sanchez, Jose E., and Johnson, Bruce D. 1986. "Women and The Drugs-Crime Connection: Crime Rates Among Drug Abusing Women At Rikers Island," *Narcotic and Drug Research*, The New York State Division of Substance Abuse, pp. 2–33.

Savitt, Todd, L. 1978. *Medicine and Slavery*. University of Illinois Press, Urbana, pp. 227–313.

Singer, A. 1974. "Mothering Practices and Heroin Addiction." *American Journal of Nursing*, vol. 74 (1), pp. 77–82.

Solomon, Kenneth. 1982. "Counseling the Drug Dependent Woman: Special Issues for Men." In *Treatment Services for Drug Dependent Women*, Reed, Buschner, and Mondanaro, eds. vol. 2. DHHS, NIDA, Washington, D.C., pp. 582–84.

Sontag, Susan. 1988. "AIDS and Its Metaphors," *New York Review of Books*, vol. 35 (16), October 27, pp. 89–99.

Spillers, Hortense J. 1985. "Interstices: A Small Drama of Words," In *Pleasures and Danger*, Vance, C., ed. Routledge and Kegan Paul, Boston, p. 73.

Stanton, Norma. 1985. Unpublished manuscript, Hispanic Women's Center, New York.

Stevens-Arroyo, Antonio M. 1980. "Puerto Rican Struggles in the Catholic Church," in *The Puerto Rican Struggle*, Rodriquez, C. E., et al., eds., Maplewood, N.J.: Waterfront Press, pp. 129–39.

Sundal-Hansen, L. Sunny. 1985. "Sex-Role Issues in Counseling Women and Men," In *Handbook of Cross-Cultural Counseling and Therapy*, Pederson, P., ed. Praeger, New York, pp. 217–19.

Tesh, Sylvia Noble. 1988. *Hidden Arguments, Political Ideology and Disease Prevention Policy*. Rutgers University Press, New Brunswick.

Tucker, M. Belinda. 1985. "U.S. Ethnic Minorities and Drug Abuse: An Assessment of Science and Practice," *International Journal of the Addictions*, vol. 20 (6 & 7), pp. 1021–47.

Vance, Carol S. 1985. "Pleasure and Danger: Toward a Politics of Sexuality," In *Pleasure and Danger*, Vance, C., ed. Routledge and Kegan Paul, Boston, pp. 8–19.

Williams, Delores S. 1985. "Black Women's Literature and the Task of Feminist Theology," In *Immaculate and Powerful*, Atkinson C. W., Buchanan C. H., and Miles, M. R., eds. Beacon Press, Boston, pp. 104–06.

Woodward, C. Vann. 1988. "Slaves and Mistresses," *New York Review of Books*, December 8, p. 3.

Worth, Dooley. 1988. "Working with Female IVDUs and Sexual Partners in New York City," NIDA Technical Review Meeting, January 19–20.

Worth, Dooley, and Rodriquez, Ruth. 1987. "Latina Women and AIDS." SIECUS Report, January-February, vol. 15 (3), pp. 5–7

Zahn, Margaret A., and Ball, John C. 1974. "Patterns and Causes of Drug Addiction among Puerto Rican Females," *Addictive Diseases: An International Journal*, vol. 1 (2), pp. 203–13.

# Chapter Nine

## Language and AIDS

### William L. Leap

## INTRODUCTION

This chapter examines the ways in which people talk about AIDS. It explores the meanings that people assign to AIDS, and to themselves in relationship to AIDS, when they participate in those discussions.

The point of view guiding this analysis builds on two of the classic claims of anthropological linguistics: Edward Sapir's comment that "language is a guide to social reality" (1949: 162), and, Benjamin Lee Whorf's observation that language patterns and cultural norms "[grow] up together, constantly influencing each other" (1956: 156). Knowledge of language and knowledge of the world are closely related phenomena, according to these statements, and the relationships which link them are in no sense accidental or arbitrary. People use language to express meanings, but they also use it to create and bestow them—particularly in instances where the topic under discussion has only recently become a part of the speakers' social experience, or for some other reason, seems to them to be unusual, irregular, or disquieting.

Hence the connection between language and AIDS. AIDS is a relatively new phenomenon for most speakers of English,[1] and, as Gilbert Herdt (1987:1) has noted, the discourse surrounding this phenomenon is *anything* but neutral. Speakers have to take both of these factors into account when they talk about AIDS or about AIDS-related themes. How they do this, and how this affects the meanings that they assign to AIDS, and to themselves in such situations, are the issues of concern in this chapter.

## NAMING THE UNNAMED

Non-neutral discourse has surrounded "the AIDS question" since the earliest days of this health crisis. Among the contributing factors were: the sudden appearance of AIDS on the international health scene; its rapid spread across national and social boundaries; the diversity and complexity of its external symptoms; the absence of effective treatment strategies; as well as the close association between occurrence of AIDS and segments of the national population already considered to be, in some sense, "non-neutral" themselves.

But also contributing to its non-neutrality, of course, was the fact that this "new disease" did not have a name. As a result, there arose "a dizzying array of acronyms . . . being banded about as possible monikers for (the) epidemic" (Shilts 1987:137), each contributing its own subtle commentary on the medical and social conditions at hand. Shilts continues:

Besides GRID (Gay Related Immune Deficiency), some doctors liked ACIDS, for Ac-quired Community Immune Deficiency Syndrome, and then others favored CAIDS, for Community Acquired Immune Deficiency Syndrome. The CDC hated GRID and pre-ferred calling it "the epidemic of immune deficiency." The "community" in other ver-sions, of course, was a polite way of saying gay; the doctors couldn't let go of the notion that one identified this disease by whom it hit rather than what it did. (Shilts 1987:158)

Doctors were not the only persons in America who identified this disease in terms of "whom it hit." From several points of view, there were advantages to be gained from "naming the unnamed" in terms of such references. For one thing, terms like GRID,[2] Gay Plague, and the like (for a detailed inventory of these terms, and discussion of the social context surrounding their use, see Murray and Payne 1988) established ownership over this health condition among persons who were not a part of the speakers' immediate experience; they made it, in other words, "somebody else's health problem," not their own. That, in turn, allowed speakers to advance a satisfying, even if somewhat self-serving explanation for the existence of AIDS: suspicious people get suspicious diseases.

Learning that this "gay disease" was also showing up among IV drug users, prostitutes, and some Caribbean blacks did not alter the logic of this argument. These were also "suspicious" populations, from the point of view of the society at large, and that made it easy to consider them as members of the same "suspect class." Reasons why persons with hemophilia were also among those at risk were obscured under this analysis—unless one simply assumed, as many did, that *all* persons with AIDS were homosexual persons.

The ready-made appeal of these "whom it hit" labels and the "comforting" point of view that they brought to any discussion of the emerging health crisis made it all the more significant that, first within the scientific community and then, though less rapidly, throughout the society as a whole, the term *AIDS* became the label-of-choice for this disease. This term does not assume that members of *any* particular group are inherently "at risk"; nor does a speaker's use of this term reinforce value-laden assumptions about the existence of the disease or the social status of those who come in contact with it.

It would be wrong, however, to conclude that *AIDS* gives speakers of English a means for overcoming the conditions of "non-neutral discourse" captured so forcefully by other, more subjective labels. Initial appearances to the contrary, *AIDS* carries with it a point of view similar to the one just described—an emphasis on the *distance* separating speaker from conditions at risk, and on the *irregular* nature of the "at risk" condition itself.

*AIDS* expresses this point of view through several means, including:

• *The combination of meanings presented by the words acquired, immunodeficiency, and syndrome*

Used by itself, *deficiency* identifies an absence of features otherwise expected to be present in a given situation. Importantly, it also implies that the situation being described has been weakened or disadvantaged, in some way, by this absence.

Absent in this case is the ability to successfully resist certain types of diseases to which, under other circumstances, human beings are typically *immune*. *Immunodeficiency* is especially serious, given that it is not an inherent condition but has become introduced into the given situation through contact with some external source; that is, the immune deficiency is *acquired*.

Importantly, the wording of this label does not make clear *why* acquisition has occurred. However, it is clear that the acquisition of immune deficiency is not an isolated event, but is something which occurs in any number of contexts—the condition is described as a syndrome. *Syndrome* is not a word commonly used during English language conversations in nontechnical contexts. And usually, when it does occur, the condition that it identifies has already been assigned less-than-desirable characteristics. *Syndrome* is an appropriate element within this term in both of these senses.

·• *The length of the construction*

"Ordinary" English—the language spoken outside of scientific, clinical, or academic domains, contains few expressions made up of sequences of three or more words. When expressions of that length do occur, the meanings of those expressions always draw attention to things distinct from the everyday experiences of speakers and listeners, to things which need to be respected (or feared) because of the special qualities associated with them. English speakers describe details of everyday experience in terms that are much less complex in structure or composition. So whatever else is implied by the meaning of this three-word phrase, reference to an *acquired immunodeficiency syndrome* cannot be a reference to an ordinary occurrence, measured in terms of this criterion.

• *Popularity of the construction's abbreviated form*

We know that "length of construction" is an issue for speakers of English in this case. Almost from the moment that *acquired immunodeficiency syndrome* became the term-of-choice in American English, speakers began to rework it into the now-familiar abbreviation: *AIDS*. Use of the abbreviation certainly made the reference process considerably less cumbersome. At the same time, reference by abbreviation establishes, through the fact of shared linguistic structure, parallels between the meaning of AIDS and the meanings of other references specified by abbreviations in American English. Those references include things that people hold in high personal regard, for example, USA, JFK, Ph.D. (particularly if it specifies one's own achievement). In those cases, the parallels do not properly apply, and use of an abbreviation highlights this contrast. The parallels are much more appropriate in instances like IRS, FBI, LSD, TB, STD (on the last usage, see comments below), where abbreviations specify references to things which the American public does not value highly, things with which most Americans prefer to have as little association as possible. Reference to AIDS via abbreviation underscores similarities with the social meanings common to items in the latter category, just as it contrasts with the social meanings in the former one. The exchange of information during discussions of AIDS cannot help but be affected by *both* of these messages.

• *The camouflaging effects of the abbreviation*

There are other advantages of the abbreviated form of this term of choice. An abbreviation, for example, may be much easier for a speaker to remember, compared to its unabbreviated counterpart; and that, in turn, may make the abbreviation easier to learn. But it becomes possible, under such circumstances, for a speaker of English to master the abbreviated form of the "correct" expression, and to use it in conversations, without being consciously aware of the full detail of the unabbreviated phrase or the precise meaning that the abbreviation has subsumed. In fact, in more than a few instances, for example, PCB (the pollutants found in electrical transformers), PCP (the hallucinogen commonly called "angel dust"), and HIV (the viral agent which causes AIDS), most speakers (and listeners) of American English would probably be hard-pressed to make such identifications accurately, were they asked to do so. Unfamiliarity with such detail does not prevent people from using those abbreviations when the topics under discussion require it. And by doing that, speakers are using terms they may not completely understand to talk about topics which are, in the sense just noted, unusual and irregular in their own right. Such a usage strategy makes its own contribution to the meaning expressed and exchanged in such discussions; that strategy becomes particularly relevant when the discussion involves a topic as disquieting as AIDS.

## ALTERNATIVE APPROACHES TO REFERENCE

Whether the speaker uses highly subjective and emotion-laden expressions like *Gay Plague* or *GRID*, or words and phrases that appear to be more objective in their presentation of meaning, the non-neutral nature of the discourse surrounding AIDS is paralleled by the non-neutral point of view which underlies the terminology of that discourse. In other words, regardless of the message that the speaker intends to be communicating, any discussion of AIDS ultimately becomes an encounter, through language, with the "irregular status" of this health condition as well as an encounter with the uncertainty which accompanies it. In other words, by talking about AIDS, the speaker is building a relationship between self and object which, under every other circumstance, the speaker would actively be seeking to avoid.

It is quite clear that some speakers of American English have no problem working in terms of such encounters and the meanings, explicit and implicit, that they contain. And in some instances, speakers actively attempt to maximize the occurrence of such language-based AIDS encounters, and to make fullest use out of the effects those encounters have on the given conversation. (I will return to this matter below.)

In other cases—and, I suspect, in the majority of instances within "ordinary English" conversations—speakers of American English adopt exactly the opposite stance. Instead of maximizing language-based encounters with AIDS, they turn to one or more of the following strategies to find ways to minimize the occurrence of such encounters, refocusing in the process the meaning of the discussion into other, "safer" domains:

• *Use open-ended references to illness*

Let the listener infer the specific illness in question from context or other clues.

Some of the generic phrases which can be used for such purposes (e.g., *he is ill, she is sick*) are much more neutral in their presentation of meaning than are others (e.g., *my buddy is bad off*). The choice of a particular generic phrase for this purpose is itself a meaningful act, and makes its own contribution to the information being expressed within the discussion. Perhaps this explains why *it*—the most open-ended and neutral of all of the English pronouns, has become such a popular replacement for direct reference to AIDS in recent months.

• *Index one or more of the external symptoms commonly associated with this disease*

For example, *She has pneumonia, He has "KS."* This option is particularly appropriate when the tone of the discussion calls on the speaker to give reasons or another explanation for a person's illness, rather than just to identify or describe it. As above, choice of symptom is itself a meaningful act, and speakers have to choose symptoms very carefully if they follow this strategy. The media and public education programs have drawn close linkages between AIDS and *pneumonia*, certain types of *cancer*, and other conditions, such that references to those conditions are automatically assumed to be a reference to AIDS, whatever the intention of the discussion.

• *Rely on synonyms and/or code words*

Use either expressions whose AIDS-related references are commonly recognized as such by society at large, or expressions which are significant only for the speaker's close associates. *Disability* is becoming widely used as a synonym for AIDS, particularly among people with AIDS, their caregivers, and their social service workers. The relative neutrality of this term is appealing—one can, after all, be disabled for any number of reasons; and so are its political implications—specifically, the obligation of public assistance programs to extend disability benefits and related services to PWAs.

Another synonym for AIDS, and one not always confined to discussions where speakers are unfamiliar with the disease, is *positive HIV status*. (I discuss *test positive*, a more colloquial variant of this expression, below.) At issue here is the outcome of a particular serological test, designed to determined whether a person has been exposed to the AIDS virus. *Positive status* refers to the presence of HIV-antibodies, evidence of previous exposure to the virus; *negative status* indicates an absence of that evidence.

From a medical point of view, it is the virus, and not AIDS itself, which is at issue in this expression. Unfortunately, some speakers of English do not always maintain this distinction between cause and consequence, and equate presence of virus with presence of AIDS. The implications of that equation can be enormous—particularly for persons who are otherwise in excellent physical and mental health and are fully committed to remaining so.

Distorted references of a second type have also become associated with the use of AIDS synonyms. In "ordinary English" usage, when the *presence* of a feature is labeled as "positive," the characteristics associated with that feature are also considered to be "positive" in basis. But in the present context, "positive" has been assigned *exactly* the opposite meaning: *presence* of feature may be labeled positive, but the attributes of the feature itself convey distinctly negative references.

Judged against those standards, the phrase *positive HIV status* contains an ambiguous, if not contradictory, set of references, consistent perhaps with the social meaning assigned to the phenomenon being described, but ambiguous and contradictory all the same. Hence it is no wonder that sentences like, *Your test came out positive*, turn out to be confusing to persons receiving their HIV test results, as well as to the person supplying the information. Multilingual and cross-cultural conversations on these themes merely intensify the possibility of such ambiguities.

*Code words* differ from *synonyms* only in that their meaning is shared among members of a particular social group and not by the larger society as a whole. The narrator and main character in a recent AIDS-related short story (Mars-Jones 1986) uses *slim* in this fashion. As he explains in the opening sentences of the story's first paragraph: "I don't use that word. I've heard it enough. So I've taken it out of circulation, just here, just at home. I say Slim instead, and Buddy understands. I have got Slim" (Mars-Jones 1986:1).

The use of highly personalized shared references, of the sort shown here, gives a group of speakers a means of indexing meanings that they have in common, while reminding themselves of the intimacy and the solidarity that they also share. Importantly, *code words* like *slim* are highly context-specific and, as such, may not be intended as reference items for the general public. Not surprisingly, an "outsider's" attempt to use *code words* in such discussions, even when prompted with sincere and sympathetic intentions, runs the risk of offending the persons the "outsider" is trying to engage.

• *Borrow words and phrases from some other dialect, language, or language tradition*

*Slim*, the code word in the Mars-Jones narrative, is also the key word in a phrase—the slim disease—widely used as a synonym for AIDS in Uganda, Kenya, and elsewhere in East Africa. That an item from East African English vernacular has now extended the vocabulary of British/American gay fiction is worth noting here. The connections between the two usage contexts would be interesting ones to explore.

*Slim* is only one of the instances where members of one language tradition have turned to the terminology from a second language tradition to find a source for their AIDS-related vocabulary. The intrusive nature of the "new" term is usually indicated quite clearly in such borrowings, often because first language pronunciation and/or grammatical detail is retained within second language setting. The symbolic value associated with such instances of linguistic "intrusion" can be quite powerful, and can communicate much in their own right— particularly if, as may be the case here of the participants in the discussion, the topic being labeled through these means is itself something "intrusive."

This is certainly what occurs, for example, during native language discussions of AIDS in American Indian communities. All American Indian languages contain mechanisms for word-building and new word creation. In fact, the "rules of speaking" in some Indian communities favor the use of these mechanisms (or the extension of existing word-meanings to cover new references) over the borrowing of terms from other languages, when Indian language conversations include attention to nontraditional themes.

In the five Indian language contexts where I have explored this matter, Indian language-based reference strategies become useful resources when speakers (or concerned outsiders) need to make indirect references to AIDS in such discussions. But when direct reference to AIDS or to an AIDS-related issue is required, speakers of those Indian languages turn to English loan words to find the necessary words and phrases. They avoid the possibilities of new word creation which their ancestral language grammars have provided to them. In fact, when AIDS becomes the topic of conversations, it is not uncommon to find Indian people shifting the whole discussion into an English language format and abandoning for the moment the use of their tribal language.

I do not think that the instances of "code-switching" or of vocabulary preference at issue here are random or arbitrary in basis. Members of most tribes tend to be nonjudgmental about the many facets of the human condition. Illness is not viewed as a punishment for sin, as is widely held in some non-Indian circles, for example, nor are personality characteristics (including details of sexual/gender orientation) considered to be evidence of weakness, shortcoming, or failure. At the same time, Indian people are quick to point out that AIDS has come into the tribal communities from outside sources, and they note that there are conflicts between those sources and the principles of "appropriate behavior" common to most Indian traditions.

Implicit in such statements, of course, is the presumed causal relationship between AIDS and homosexual behavior. Also present here is the belief, erroneously based (see Williams 1987 for details) though widely held in some Indian and non-Indian circles all the same, that "gay" behavior is not traditional to the tribal experience in native North America, and that "gay Indians" exist today only because the "corrupting" influence of the surrounding, non-Indian society.

The social "benefits" implicit in both of these points of view are considerable. By classifying AIDS as something "intrusive," and deriving AIDS from external sources already known to have inflicted great damage on Indian well-being, Indian people are able to account for the presence of the health crisis while minimizing their own members' involvement, as actors, in the conditions of that crisis. (This is, of course, the same thing non-Indians do when they label AIDS as a "gay disease" or account for the pandemic by citing the African origin of the virus.) Reference to AIDS through English language terms, rather than Indian ones, is entirely consistent with the "we" vs. "they" dichotomy implicit in such discussions; moreover, it gives Indians a way of representing that position quite vividly, regardless of audience, each time this matter is discussed.

• *Use medical, technical, clinical, or other scientific jargon instead of "ordinary English"*

The linguistic process at issue here is similar to the ones described under the preceding category. However, the linguistic items and the perspective on meaning that they introduce into the discussion is quite distinct. Instead of highlighting the socially accepted meanings of AIDS, this strategy lets speakers obscure these meanings, even if they do so in a publically acceptable, quite elegant fashion.

Described in these terms, a person does not just "get AIDS." Rather, he or she is "exposed to the retrovirus" and, after several months, "undergoes seroconversion"; then, after a "latency period" of anywhere from six months to perhaps twenty years in duration, he or she begins to exhibit certain combinations of symptoms, suggesting the presence of one or more "opportunistic infections" or other evidence of underlying cellular "immunodeficiency." It is that evidence which confirms the presence of AIDS.

For some speakers of English, "exposed to the retrovirus," "seroconversion," and other forms of technical vocabulary take the discussion of AIDS out of the realm of ordinary experience and assign it a "special status." Both of these are outcomes which these speakers are consciously seeking to avoid, and not surprisingly, they resist using such terminology whenever they talk about these themes. (What they say, and how they phrase it, that is, the vocabulary and grammar of AIDS in "ordinary English," needs to be the subject of a separate chapter.)

For others, however, the descriptive precision and other components of reference through technical vocabulary carry a certain appeal. Hence recent efforts designed to strengthen public awareness about AIDS use these terms throughout their discussions, as do the articles on AIDS found in the scientific literature and, frequently, in the popular journals. Clinical vocabulary provides the terms of choice for discussions of AIDS issues by public health authorities and case-workers. Often, this is the idiom of discourse when practitioners, care-givers, and people with AIDS interact. Clinical vocabulary, in other words, constitutes the central core of an emerging "standard language" of AIDS in America. These are the terms that speakers of English *should* use if they wish to talk about AIDS "correctly."

Some of these clinically based, "standard language" expressions have begun to appear within "ordinary language" conversations, thanks to aggressive public education programs. Whether speakers will use the terms "correctly" under these circumstances (that is, maintain the reference focus found within technical, clinical domains, even though the context of discussion has changed) is another matter entirely. The frequent confusion of *HIV-positive status* with *AIDS* itself, discussed above, is one example of the type of misunderstanding which can occur under such circumstances.

And even when used in clinical contexts, the technical, specialized vocabulary at issue in this strategy may lead to unintended reference consequences. Some of these are shown in the recent (1988) revisions of the "universal blood and bodily fluid precautions" in the *Precaution Manual* of a large public hospital in the northeastern United States. These revisions allowed the text of the manual to take into account risk factors associated with the treatment of persons with AIDS who, in increasing numbers, are now seeking outpatient services as well as long-term care through this facility. The revised *purpose* and *rationale* of this section of the manual reads as follows:

PURPOSE: To prevent transmission of communicable disease in the health care setting.

RATIONALE: The increasing prevalence of Human Immunodeficiency Virus (HIV) and Hepatitis B (HBV) increases the likelihood that health care workers will be exposed to blood from patients infected with those viruses. Authorities now recommend that health care workers consider *all* patients as potentially infected with HIV, HBV, and/or other blood-borne pathogens. Universal blood and body fluid precautions are recommended to minimize this risk.

Even though, according to comments from the hospital staff, the AIDS epidemic prompted these revisions, references to *AIDS* do not occur at *any* point in the new text. *HIV* is mentioned in several places, but always in conjunction with references to *HBV* (hepatitis B virus) and other "blood-borne pathogens." The similarities between the "pathogens" implied by this listing does little to draw attention to the particular risks facing health care professionals in AIDS/ HIV-related treatment contexts or to the *specific* strategies they should follow in order to minimize those risks. Indeed, taken on face value, it is difficult to determine whether this portion of the procedures manual has anything to do with *AIDS* at all. And that may be the biggest problem growing out of discussions of *AIDS* couched in technical, clinical vocabulary.

• *Adopt the reference strategies which describe sexually transmitted diseases (STDs)*

This approach to AIDS reference differs in several ways from the other approaches to AIDS reference that are being discussed here. Most important, perhaps, is its basis in words, phrases, and expressions which have already become familiar to members of American society, thanks to recent efforts to increase public awareness about chlamydia, herpes, gonorrhea, syphilis, and the other diseases within this category. In the mid–1970s, public health officials began using *sexually transmitted diseases*, commonly abbreviated *STDs*, as a general label for these conditions. Among other benefits, this usage allowed public health workers to refer to these diseases under a single, inclusive heading, while avoiding the negative associations connected to *veneral disease*, their more traditional cover-term.

Along with the new label came two other things: 1) a set of stock phrases, which gave speakers new ways to refer to these themes, and 2) a more open, and supportive attitude toward the subject matter which encouraged people to talk directly and freely about them.

Taken on face value, this reference strategy and the ideas it represents can be quite functional in an AIDS discussion. The topics are parallel in many ways, and so is the language which must be used to discuss them. Note, for example, how the following statement from a pamphlet prepared by the American College Health Association could, with no major adjustment in wording, introduce a pamphlet advising college students of the dangers of *AIDS*.

Sexually transmitted diseases (STDs), formerly known as VD (veneral disease), are diseases that are acquired through sexual contact. Many people think of gonorrhea and syphilis as the only STDs, while in reality there are probably more than 20 STDs. Some people think that only dirty or promiscuous people get STDs but that is not true. No one is immune to STDs, but those with multiple partners or many casual sex partners are at increased risk of developing an STD. (ACHA 1985:2)

And similarly, the following suggestions for avoiding STD infection constitute appropriate AIDS-avoidance strategies:

First, do not have sexual relations with someone who has an STD, and try to avoid having intercourse with someone who has more than one sexual partner. A condom can offer excellent protection against many sexually transmitted diseases. There is evidence that vaginal spermacides (foam, jelly) may help kill some STD organisms. . . . However, should you have any reason to suspect that you have contracted an STD, do yourself and your partner a favor—seek medical treatment. (ACHA 1985:2)

So it is not surprising to find speakers of American English using words and phrases common to STD reference contexts when talking about AIDS. Parallels in reference are quite easy to construct in most instances. That is, just as someone *gets the clap*, so he or she *gets AIDS*. The process of transmission—intimate sexual contact with a person who already has the disease—is the same in both instances, and so is the verb (*get*) which is used to describe that process. A self-diagnosis may be possible once the individual becomes familiar with the external symptoms, but self-diagnosis is never reliable and often misleading and ultimately laboratory analysis (commonly referred to as *the test* in both instances) is needed in order to confirm the presence of the disease-causing pathogen.

Classifying AIDS as an STD has its limitations, however. Public confidence in the availability (and effectiveness) of treatment of diseases traditionally in-cluded under the label STD has, in some instances, led people to have "positive contact" with one or more carriers of these diseases, then to transmit that condition through sexual activity with one or more previously uninfected per-sons, then to seek diagnosis and receive treatment, and then to become infected with another STD once again—all within a relatively brief period of time.

The public health related implications of such behavior are considerably more serious when AIDS, rather than syphilis or gonorrhea, is the STD being transmitted through these encounters. Unfortunately, however, the same sort of preference for high frequency, multiple-partnered, cyclical sexual encounters, accompanied by a disregard for the long-term consequences of such actions, was very much a part of the early days of the AIDS health crisis and is still in evidence today in spite of recent, intensified efforts at public health education. Of course we can explain the presence of such encounters within the context of the pandemic by citing the participants' commitment to needs-centered, selfish sexual gratification. But a thorough analysis of the social dynamics of the AIDS health crisis will want to determine whether assumptions about the avail-ability of treatment for other STDs are in any sense being applied here; that is, stating the matter directly, if you can *get AIDS* like you *get the clap*, then you should be able to *cure AIDS* like you can *cure the clap*. Parallels in linguistic features, particularly verb structures, certainly provide a structural basis for such analogies.

## A GENERAL RULE: DISCUSS THE ISSUE BUT AVOID THE NAME

Thus far, this chapter has described some of the ways in which speakers of American English refer to AIDS. Each of these options allows English speakers to give a distinct focus to the issues under discussion, by letting them highlight certain themes while downplaying or distracting attention from others. The range of options and varieties of points of view expressed by them are the critical elements here. People who *listen* to talk about AIDS—whether the comments come from politicians, researchers, persons from the news media, concerned laypersons, friends and family members of persons with AIDS, as well as persons with AIDS themselves—need to be aware that these options exist, and that a speaker's use of one of them is closely tied to the speaker's point of view on AIDS issues as a whole.

It is, however, necessary to acknowledge the several areas in which all of these reference strategies have similar effects on discussions of AIDS–differences in speaker point of view notwithstanding. For example, it is important to note how almost every one of the strategies cited here give speakers of English ways to talk about AIDS *without* mentioning the topic by name. The symbolic value of such omissions is powerful, especially given the "irregular" meanings already assigned to this health condition and to those persons associated with it. There is no better way for a speaker of English to maintain distance from such a topic, than by talking about it exclusively through indirect references.[3]

Of course any number of misunderstandings can arise when communication is structured in these terms. For instance, speaker A, who has not seen speaker B for some time, may open a conversations by saying, "Hey, you've lost weight." That remark could have no underlying agenda (other than, perhaps, just a hint of jealousy), though it could be intended as a coded inquiry into the AIDS-related status of speaker B's health. The statement could be interpreted, and responded to, in either of these senses by speaker B, whatever speaker A's intent, thereby increasing the likelihood of miscommunication. So it is not surprising to find that pointed comments about another person's weight, dietary habits, complexion, and the like are no longer considered to be appropriate remarks during casual conversation, particularly by persons who consider themselves to be "at risk" from the epidemic and choose to mark this status through language choice.

## THE SOCIAL SIGNIFICANCE OF DIRECT REFERENCE

Earlier in this chapter, I noted that some speakers of English appear not to have difficulty with *AIDS* references and will, accordingly, mention AIDS by name whenever they find it appropriate to do so. Having looked at the "rules" and reference strategies which promote the avoidance of this term, we are now ready to consider the conditions under which speakers of American English bypass these alternative ways of referring to AIDS and mention AIDS directly by name.

As might be expected, direct references often occur in clinical or medical settings; certainly they are prompted by the discussions that occur within those domains. Even so, the message that accompanies direct references in such contexts should not be treated lightly. A willingness to use the term *AIDS* when discussing his or her own health status or health-related concerns within a clinical context suggests that the individual has had some level of success in coming to terms with the health crisis and its impact on all of our lives. This person's attitude about AIDS should be different from that of a person who uses generic references, or other reference strategies in such situations. And if this person continues to make direct references to AIDS in conversational settings outside of clinical or medical contexts, the prediction about AIDS-acceptance becomes more powerfully confirmed.

At the other extreme, however, are those instances where direct reference to AIDS has nothing to do with the speaker's (or the listener's) physical or mental well-being, but where comments are made for shock value, as part of some larger, attention-getting strategy, or merely to reflect the extent of one's own awareness of "the current scene."

At issue here are motion picture reviews which claim that the underlying theme of a commercially popular film like *Fatal Attraction* is AIDS-retaliation, not the destructive consequences of marital infidelity on *all* parties to the affair; or to treat the ever-expanding, inexplicable protoplasm in the summer 1988 film *The Blob* as a visual metaphor for the AIDS virus itself. Also at issue here are children's taunts on playgrounds and in shopping malls, "You have a cold, I bet you're gonna get AIDS," and the ever-growing number of AIDS-jokes which let adults attempt to make "sick humor" out of the most basic conditions of the health crisis. Speculation in the news media's obituaries regarding the "real cause of death" (and, by extension, the sexual preferences) of politicians, movie stars, entertainers, and other famous persons certainly falls within this category, as do segments within several of Eddie Murphy's films.

One of the more serious by-products of such usages is the trivialization that it gives to AIDS issues. Repeated, casual comment on *any* topic makes it difficult for listeners to treat that topic seriously, particularly if the comments take the form of unplanned, off-handed remarks, or if they associate discussions of AIDS with discussions of nonserious themes. Such is frequently the presentation given to the AIDS health crisis in the media commentaries, talk show programming, "pulp" newspapers and supermarket "scandal sheets," and in other "commercialized" and "popular" news/entertainment materials. Anyone can be a quotable authority on AIDS in these contexts, and any connection with AIDS, regardless of its long-term value, deserves its share of public attention. Unfortunately, in the absence of more broadly based, publicly supported programs of AIDS education, people have to turn to such materials to find answers to their questions about AIDS. What they learn from these sources does not always advance the national interests in AIDS-related health education; that is another danger associated with trivialization.

## IMPLICATIONS FOR THE REFERENCE TO "SELF"

Having looked at some of the ways in which people talk about AIDS, and the meanings that accompany the speaker's use of each of those options, we are now ready to explore another dimension of the relationship between language and AIDS—how speakers use language to establish their sense of self,[4] as actor and/or as observer, within AIDS related social domains.

"Self" can be expressed through language by any number of means. I propose to examine the effects two of those options—choice of verb reference and choice of personal pronoun—have on the presentation of self in AIDS-related discussions.

## Choice of Verb Reference

The verb is the component of a sentence which specifies the action undertaken by the sentence subject, or the action with which the subject is otherwise involved. Verbs are critical elements in the grammar of all English sentences, and the speaker's choice of verb usually has a profound effect on the meaning which that sentence maintains.

For example, a speaker of English could use any one of the following constructions[5] to describe his or her health status:

1. I caught AIDS.
2. I got AIDS.
3. I've come down with AIDS.
4. I have AIDS.

But note how the meaning of these sentences varies considerably, example by example, and how differences in meaning signaled by the sentence verb has a lot to do with this variation.

To illustrate this point, let's look briefly at the contrasts in meaning maintained by two of these examples. The message presented in sentence (1) is quite straightforward. Sentence subject is the *receiver* of sentence action. In order for the subject to *catch* something, the item in question must be based (for the moment, at least) outside of the person's control. Moreover, some other party, acting independently of the intended recipient, has to initiate the process of transmission; most likely that person will assume responsibility for the event, or be blamed for it, once transmission is completed.

The sentence subject in this example, the person who "caught" AIDS, has to be specified in sentence structure, in order to have a grammatically acceptable construction. The constraints on the reference to any other party involved in this transaction are somewhat more flexible. That is, the other party may be listed by name in the sentence (*I caught AIDS from my roommate*), designated indirectly through an association with place, time, or process of transmission (*I caught AIDS during last summer's vacation*), or simply acknowledged through the assumptions about "cause" implicit in the verb reference (If I caught AIDS, I must have caught it from someone—a good example of the use of conversational implicature cited in Note 3).

Importantly, whatever option the speaker selects, the *source* of the illness remains at a distance from the party who ultimately encounters it when *catch* is selected as the sentence verb. Similarly, sentences with *have* as the main verb, as in sentence (4), say nothing about the extent of the subject's involvement in the transmission process. Here, however, the parallels end. For unlike *catch* sentences, *have* sentences do not make any explicit comment on the reason for action, nor do they provide clues regarding implicit causality. Reference to the time of the event and other details of context are also minimized in such sentences. Note the use of the "neutral" present tense on the verb in sentence (4), in contrast to the explicit past tense reference in sentence (1). In fact, *have* sentences highlight only the fact of relationship connecting sentence subject (*I* in this case) and sentence object (*AIDS* in this case).

Of course, the listener is free to draw whatever inferences he or she wants to make regarding the reason(s) for the relationship or the persons responsible for it. But the simplicity of information contained within sentence structure in this case suggests that the fact of relationship between subject and verb—and, specifically in this case, between speaker and AIDS—is the intended centerpiece of this reference. At least, this is the centerpiece that the speaker's verb choice appears to be highlighting.

## Choice of Personal Pronoun

Choices between pronouns provide speakers with another means for describing their "place" within AIDS-related reference contexts, and of specifying how their participation in some AIDS-related event coincides or conflicts with the activities of other, involved parties.

Consider, for example, the differences in pronoun usage in the following two passages, each of which presents an IV drug user's description of his or her "needle-sharing" behavior in Seattle.[6] Note the differences in meanings and speaker "sense of self" which the speaker's choice of pronoun calls to mind in each case:

## Speaker: A

Passage A-1

*Question:* Did you share needles?

*Answer:* Yes, I did.

*Question:* When would you share needles?

*Answer:* I basically had my own needles. I'd share with other people that would come in and want to buy drugs and if I were out of points that I was selling and they wanted to be hit up or something, you know, I'd always rinse the point, rinse the needle and tell them that it was used, it was mine and tell them that they were taking their chances.

**Speaker: B**

Passage B–1

*Question:* Can you describe a typical needle sharing situation?

*Answer:* Yeah. We'd cop, just use the same spoons, the same cotton, the same everything. And, uh, we'd use the same needle.

*Question:* How many people would be using the same needle?

*Answer:* Ordinarily, I was using used needles already. There would be three of us shooting but I'd just be in situations where you just used whatever outfit came through the door. And it was probably used the next room over, and, uh, there was no cleaning of it, there was no nothing. I mean sometimes there'd be times where, where we loaded up and it'd be go half, I mean, the guy would plunge and do half of the needle and then I'd do the rest. It'd be from one arm to another. Every time was different.

Speaker A bases his comments on a rhetorical contrast between "self" and "others" and he uses the distinction between actions involving *I* and actions involving *they* as a means of presenting that contrast to the listener. *I* has needles to share, and will let others use them. *I* always made an effort to clean the point before giving it to someone else, and *I* warned *them* that the needle had already been used and "they were taking their chances." *They* are the persons "at risk" in this exchange, according to the wording that the speaker gives to this passage: *they* are using needles which *I* knows have been used before, and *I* makes a point of telling *them*, in advance, that *they* are putting *themselves* at risk through *their* action.

Nowhere in this passage does the speaker acknowledge that he placed himself in any danger through his needle-sharing. The *I* vs. *they* dichotomy, indexed so neatly through the pronoun contrasts which recur throughout the passage and the emphasis on a one-way (e.g., *I* to *they*) transfer of needles across that dichotomy keeps the speaker's references to self neatly detached from his references to danger. It also separates him from any responsibility for the "conditions of risk" presented to other parties as a result of these transactions; he warned them, in advance, that the needles were used and they were "taking their chances."

The speaker in the passage B–1 also described needle-sharing as a group-centered activity. But here *we*, not *I* vs. *they*, is the centerpiece for the commentary, and this makes the comments on needle-sharing presented in this passage quite different from those found in passage A–1.

As before, *I* references occur with some frequency in the narrative. Here, however, *I* identifies a subset of a larger and more inclusive *we* grouping, not a party acting independently from it. The risk of transmission of the AIDS virus is just as real here as in passage A–1. This time, instead of presenting himself as someone detached from the given conditions, *I* admits to being both coparticipant and cocontributor to that situation.

The differences in these speakers' choice of pronoun—and the contrasts in description of self which stem from each speaker's pronoun choices—are in large part reflections of certain facts about each speaker's life within the Seattle drug "community." The speaker in passage A–1 was, for a time, a supplier of drugs and the persons participating in the needle-sharing events described in his passage are clients, and not necessarily personal friends. The relationships between the participants in needle-sharing as described in passage B–1 are completely different. The group includes both friends—"there would be three of us"—as well as complete strangers—"you just used whatever outfit came through the door." Here, mutual interest in "staying high" created a common bond between participants which was quite distinct from the more commercially based, and more individualized, exchanges at issue in passage A–1.

Importantly, speaker A's choice of pronouns, and the description those choices give to his own actions as an IV drug user, alters only slightly when the speaker begins to describe needle-sharing with friends:

## Speaker: A

### Passage A–2

*Question:* Would you use needles with a group of people?

*Answer:* No. I would share my needles basically if I knew the person. I shared with the people that I know of, that I remember that I shared my needles with.

*Question:* What was your reluctance about sharing needles?

*Answer:* Fear of AIDS. These were basically people that I ran with, hung out with, dealt with.

Comments in Passage A–2 center almost exclusively around *I* references. The presence of "other participants" in the events being described is acknowledged, yet the speaker never used a *they* to refer to them. Nor, in spite of the fact that needle-*sharing* is the activity at issue here, does speaker A ever use *we* to identify the persons involved in that transaction. As in passage A–1, the speaker presents the self as an independent actor, separated and detached from the surrounding social environment, even though (as a dealer) speaker A was very much a key player within that environment. Hence there is a considerable amount of significance subsumed within the meaning of his statement, "I would share my needles basically if I knew the person": it is the relationship of the "person" to "I" which takes him/her out of the speaker's *they* reference category and minimizes the risk of contracting AIDS.

The differences in descriptions of self-as-actor which grow out of these contrasts in pronoun usage allow us to predict, among other things, that speakers A and B will evidence very different approaches to health maintenance and self-healing, once they became aware of their HIV-positive status. Such is precisely the case, according to the comments made during their interviews.

Importantly for present purposes, these differences are also reflected directly in each speaker's pronoun choices.

## Speaker: A

### Passage A–3

*Question:* What sources (of AIDS information) do you trust the most?

*Answer:* I would tend to trust my own intuition on the whole thing, you know. What I do know about it and, you know, there's doctors that say "catch the virus and you're going to die." There's no way of saving your life. But there is, if you are willing to change and if you are willing to believe. If you truly love yourself and truly believe you can heal yourself, I believe you can. Whereas, I don't think a lot of doctors are willing, you know, they can't put any documentation down.

*Question:* Do you do any other kinds of self-help practices?

*Answer:* Just do meditation and I'm going to try a diet that a friend of mine told me about. I think it has a lot to do with, you know any thing'll work if you truly believe in it. It is up to the person and their willingness to change. If they truly want to change their life and to live.

## Speaker: B

### Passage B–2

*Question:* How . . . has your life changed? How do you view your life differently? What's the process?

*Answer:* The process has been difficult because I've continued to get sicker. I mean, at first I was positive, positive with some symptoms. Then I went to ARC, then debilitating ARC, then I went to AIDS. And that, that has been a slow process for me. I don't have a lot of energy. I've been pretty sick. . . . (AIDS) is a pretty painful disease to have. And the thing is, you just never know. I mean I go like this and then down, and sometimes I go up a little bit. I am on AZT now; that helps me neurologically, too.

I have a real strong recovery program. I think that if I hadn't had Narcotics Anonymous, and I hadn't had some program behind me when I found out, I probably wouldn't have come back. I probably would have stayed out, shooting dope. I probably would have shared needles and I probably wouldn't have cared.

But I found out a year into my recovery and I watched, I mean I have a number of friends who have died of AIDS and I have sat and watched them die, and I have held their hands and I have cried . . . and I have some role models, people who are doing it (i.e., recovering), but not many people are that willing and that ready to try to change their life completely. It does take a lot; it is not easy getting clean.

*Question:* What is most important to you right now?

*Answer:* Feeling comfortable with myself, loving myself, um, recovering, trying to help other people not get into this situation, supporting people in recovery. I go to hospitals and I talk to people who are finding out they have AIDS[7] at the same time that they just OD'd. Try to tell them that if they want to come to the meeting I'd take them; if they want recovery it is there. There are people who will support them—that kind of stuff, quality of life.

As before, speaker A's statements are constructed around a distinctive and self-contained *I*, who acts independently of the social circumstances in which he lives. And as before, the underlying theme of this speaker's commentary involves an *I vs. they* contrast, even though, in this passage, instead of distinguishing between "self" and "clients," the *I vs. they* contrast now distinguishes the speaker from members of the medical profession.

Passage A–3 also contains an abundance of open-ended *you* references. Their presence is important here, since *you* is not a frequently occurring pronoun option within these interviews. When *you* does occur, it is found in conjunction with context-detached, generalized comments, whose meaning is then expanded, and made more concrete, by a series of anecdotal, personalized *I* references. *I vs. you* in this case indicates a pairing, and not a dichotomy or a contrast; contrary to first impression, the alternation between open-ended *you* and personalized *I* is the closest speaker A comes to paralleling speaker B's use of inclusive *we*.

Reference to speaker A as a singular, independent actor, was evidenced quite clearly in passages A–1 and A–2, above, and it continues to be evidenced here. This time, the reference takes on even greater personal significance. Healing, he says, is something which only *I* can do. It involves his coming to terms with himself: "anything'll work if you truly believe in it, it is up to the person and their willingness to change."

Speaker B's comments about healing also begin with speaker-centered references, and it is clear that the struggle to maintain health is both painful and demanding. Having established that point, she then expands the discussion of the healing *process* to take other parties and their physical and mental well-being into account. Speaker B acknowledges the effects that Narcotics Anonymous and numerous individual "role models" have had on her outlook on living; they appear to have been the inspiration for her own work with people with AIDS who are also struggling with these concerns.

For speaker B, healing is anything but a self-centered, socially independent process. Just as she was only one of many persons involved in IV drug use and needle-sharing, so she is only one of the many actors involved in the healing process. Her sense of self remains closely linked to her sense of the larger social group of which she is a part; her choice of pronouns, and other uses of language, makes this commitment explicitly clear.

## CONCLUSIONS

The discussion in this chapter has focused on language, particularly about the ways language choices contribute to the creation of meaning and the exchange of meaning within particular social settings. The action here is ongoing on two levels: there is meaning which grows out of the speakers' *use* of language (e.g., the selection of words and phrases, choices between options in grammar and style). And there is also meaning within the structure of language itself, whose influence on conversation and communication the speaker may be able either to highlight or to mask, but will never be able completely to submerge.

Hence, as discussed in the first sections of this chapter, there is a paradox surrounding the term *AIDS*. Use of this expression is certainly preferable to many of the other labels for this health condition, yet favoring it over those other options (a conscious decision, in most cases) does not exempt the discussion—or the speakers participating within them, from the "package" of meanings already associated with the individual words out of which this term is composed, established through its combination of words, cued through by its frequent occurrence as an abbreviation, and the like. No wonder, then, that so many different paraphrases for *AIDS* have become a part of "ordinary English" in recent years, each of which, as we have seen, adds to the references being assigned to this disease in American society, while it reinforces the complex of references already assigned there.

Speakers may not always be conscious of these options, or of their implication for meaning and reference under these circumstances. But conscious or not, they structure the content of AIDS discussions in terms of these contrasts, and structure the "grammar" of these discussions—specifically, as we have seen here, choice of verb form and pronoun—along similar lines. There are, in other words, abundant clues to speaker's point of view about AIDS and about self in relation to AIDS, to be found in the language of discussion, each time discussion occurs on these themes.

Linguists, particularly those concerned with the interaction of language and context, and the interrelationship of language and experience, writ large, can find much to interest them in the study of language and AIDS. But the issues discussed in this chapter are equally important for the interests of health care professionals and others involved in the delivery of medical and social services during the AIDS health crisis. These examples constitute the beginnings of what can become a profile of *expectable language usage* whenever speakers of American English talk about AIDS. Developing this profile can help practitioners understand more clearly and more efficiently the messages that underlie the comments and responses given by *all* parties to such discussions. Reference to this profile may also alert practitioners to the existence of problematic conditions, ranging from the self-induced hypochondria of the "worried well" to the earliest stages of AIDS-related *dementia*, long before formal diagnosis of such conditions may have been established.

Of course, the data-base needs to be expanded to take into account any number of additional variables. Most important in that regard are the wide range of factors which always lead to variability in language usage, whatever the issue under discussion. Sex and gender, region, socioeconomic status, as well as home language background are some of these factors. What we will learn from those studies will greatly enrich the descriptive power of the profile begun here and, I am confident, will add significantly to its value.

## NOTES

My thanks to Sue-Ellen Jacobs (Women's Studies and Anthropology, University of Washington, Seattle), Jeanne Kleyn (director, AIDS-IVDM Study, Alcohol and Drug Abuse Institute, University of Washington, Seattle), Charlton Clay and Tambi Shaw (Project staff members) for encouraging me in this analysis, letting me use their interview tapes and transcripts to test and refine my claims, and for taking time to read and comment on the first draft of this text.

I also acknowledge the helpful suggestions from Brett Williams, Geoff Burkhart, Naomi Baron, and Robert Morasky (The American University, Washington, DC), Michael Quam (Sangamon State University, Springfield, IL), Gilbert Herdt (University of Chicago, IL), Dana Winkler (New School for Social Research, New York City, NY), Stephen O. Murray (San Francisco, CA), and Douglas A. Feldman (University of Miami, FL).

1. The examples explored in this chapter come from discussions of AIDS by speakers of American English. The uses of language and the treatment of AIDS-related themes which the examples illustrate are not necessarily unique to the United States or to any of its social segments or speech communities.

2. I follow accepted linguistic practice here and identify the linguistic terms of interest to the discussion by underlying them within the text; hence GRID and Gay Plague in the sentence above. This allows me to distinguish between AIDS, the disease, and AIDS, one of several labels which speakers of American English use when referring to it.

3. Grice (1975 and elsewhere) uses the term conversational implicature to refer to the linguistic process at issue here. Briefly described, the implicature process allows speakers to pack a large amount of meaning into a small amount of conversational space. They do this, among other means, by regularly drawing on implicitly stated references, as often as they do explicitly stated ones, through the discussion. I am aware of few topics where Grice's claims about the impact of implicature on the success of the discourse process have been so graphically displayed.

4. The term self as used in this discussion refers to an individual's perceptions of his or her own uniqueness, as a person, where perceptions are based on assessments of one's own actions within social and cultural context(s) on the reactions others have to one's actions, and on other social, cultural considerations. Importantly, self is not a static category but a construct, continually being shaped and modified by the individual in question.

5. Other English verbs, in addition to caught, got, and have, can be used to make similar, verb-related distinctions in reference perspective and other points of contrast—person of sentence subject, verb tense, and the like—have similar effects on sentence references. Unfortunately, a more detailed description of the relationship between AIDS and the English "verbs of illness" cannot be presented here.

6. Sharing improperly cleaned needles is one of the primary ways through which the human immunodeficiency virus is transmitted among IV drug users. Obtaining detailed, first-hand descriptions of the needle-sharing process has been of great importance to the

University of Washington's intervention ethnography project, from whose bank of interviews the following passages were selected.

7. Note how differently this sentence would read, and how greatly the meaning would shift, if the speaker had used *caught* or *got*, in place of the more open-ended, subject-centered, and less inherently judgmental *have*, as the verb in this expression.

## REFERENCES

American College Health Association. 1985. Sexually transmitted diseases. Rockville, Md: Health Information Series, American College Health Association.

Grice, H.P. 1975. Logic and Conversation. In *Syntax and Semantics 3: Speech Acts*, pp. 41–58, P. Cole and J.L. Morgan, eds. New York City: Academic Press.

Herdt, Gilbert. 1987. AIDS and anthropology. *Anthropology Today* 3: 1–3.

Mars-Jones, Adam. 1986. Slim. In *The Darker Proof: Stories from a Crisis*, pp. 1–10, Edmund White and Adam Mars Jones, eds. New York: New American Library.

Murray, Stephen O., and Kenneth W. Payne. 1988. The social classification of AIDS in American epidemiology. *Medical Anthropology* 10 (2–3): 1–14.

Sapir, Edward. 1929. The Status of Linguistics as a Science. In *Selected Writings of Edward Sapir*, pp. 160–66, David Mandelbaum, ed. Berkeley: University of California Press.

Shilts, Randy. 1987. *And The Band Played On*. New York: Viking Penguin, Inc.

Whorf, Benjamin Lee. 1956. The Relation of Habitual Thought and Behavior to Language. In *Language, Thought and Reality: Selected Writings of Benjamin Lee Whorf*, pp. 134–59, John Carrol, ed. Cambridge: MIT Press.

Williams, Walter L. 1987. *The Spirit and the Flesh: Sexual Diversity in American Indian Culture*. Boston: Beacon Press.

# Chapter Ten

## AIDS and Obituaries: The Perpetuation of Stigma in the Press

Peter M. Nardi

How the general population reacts to AIDS is partly related to how it is depicted in the media. How it is portrayed in the media is a function of the stigma attached to the disease itself and to the people at highest risk in getting AIDS. What results is a socially constructed picture of illness and disease, morality and stigma, couched in a language which conceals meanings while creating new ones in their place. In other words, because of confounding concepts of morality and medicine, the media reports AIDS using language that perpetuates the stigma attached to it and to the people dying from it. As evidence of this process, this chapter investigates obituaries and their role in socially constructing meanings about AIDS.

### INTRODUCTION

Just as homosexuality was becoming demedicalized—that is, no longer perceived as a medical illness but as an alternative set of natural behaviors—AIDS enters to reinforce the connection between disease and sexuality. As Conrad and Schneider (1980) argue, many forms of deviant behavior have been defined as immoral, sinful, or criminal. But as social conditions changed, so too did definitions about deviance. What formerly were labeled as moral weaknesses, eventually were talked about as illnesses or diseases. Medicine emerged as the agent of social control, not the church or police.

These changing definitions of deviance are "treated as products of a political process, as social constructions usually implemented and legitimated by powerful and influential interests and applied to relatively powerless and subordinate

groups" (Conrad and Schneider, 1980: 36). The medicalization of deviant behavior is clearly illustrated in the definitions imposed on sexuality (in particular,
masturbation and homosexuality) throughout the nineteenth century, just as
religious prohibitions were becoming less powerful agents of control.

But unlike other forms of variant behavior, homosexuality in the post-World
War II years has been shedding its medical label. From the Kinsey studies in
the late 1940s, through the rise of gay liberation and the changes in the diagnostic manuals used by the American Psychiatric Association, homosexual behavior has been in the process of becoming demedicalized and depathologized.

Still, a stigma remains to being gay and engaging in homosexual relations.
Goffman (1963:4), for example, discusses various types of stigma, in particular,
stigma based on "blemishes of individual character" and stigma based on "abom-
inations of the body—the various physical deformities." Homosexuality is given
as an example of the first kind. With the physical deformities attributed to
AIDS, one can argue that it is an example of the second kind. Since two-thirds
of American AIDS cases are homosexual or bisexual men, being diagnosed with
AIDS is like taking on two stigmas in the public's eye: a physical deformity and
a defect in character. AIDS reintroduces medical labels and moral weaknesses
to account for its high incidence among gay men. A similar argument could be
made about the stigma attached to being an intravenous drug user.

What we are seeing, then, is the social construction of definitions and labels
to explain a complex set of behaviors and characteristics often viewed as stigmatized. Conrad and Schneider (1980: 36) state the thesis succinctly:

Illness, like deviance, is a social construction based on social judgment of some condition
in the world. Although based partly on current cultural conceptions of what constitutes
disease, and (in Western societies) typically grounded in biophysiological phenomena,
the social evaluative process of classifying some condition or event as a disease is central
rather than peripheral to the concept of disease and illness. In this fundamental sense
a disease designation is a moral judgment, for to define something as a disease or illness
is to deem it undesirable.

To be designated a "person with AIDS" is to carry a double stigma: the disease
itself and the possibility of being a gay man. In a medicalized era, these are
both viewed as illnesses, and thereby moral weaknesses. As such, AIDS is seen
as something brought on oneself due to poor character, bad judgment, and a
sick life-style (see Sontag, 1978). Albert (1986a: 167) argues that the occurrence
of AIDS overlays "an undisputed illness on a highly disputed behavior that
carries with it three judgmental options: alternative lifestyle, illness, or deviance.
AIDS presents a situation in which the physiological problem occasions the
reaffirmation of one of these already-held conceptions concerning the nature of
homosexuality."

Constructing AIDS in these terms, thus, leads to the concealment of it by
many in everyday life. To publicly acknowledge it is to take on dual stigmatized

labels that risk exposure as a weak and sick person in the public's mind. "Coming out" as a person with AIDS is not unlike "coming out" as a gay person: both involve identity issues, labeling, and the reconstruction of interaction with others. For many, these risks are too much, even after death, as illustrated by the media problem of reporting obituaries.

## THE MEDIA AND AIDS

How people construct and interpret reality is related to language. Language provides the categories and ordered meanings for experiencing the world around us, or as Berger and Luckmann (1966: 68) state it: "Language objectivates the shared experiences and makes them available to all within the linguistic community. . . . Language provides the means for objectifying new experiences." Such is the case with AIDS as it increasingly affects our social institutions and the language we use to deal with the changes in society. This is especially true when stigmas are involved, as evidenced by the language and methods used by the media in dealing with the AIDS epidemic.

Albert (1986a: 167) says that, "The media portrayals of AIDS reflect the confusion and ambiguity experienced by the society at large." He found that media coverage tended to reaffirm the stigmatized status of those at high risk: intravenous drug users and, especially, gay men. Reports emphasized deviant life-styles, thereby establishing a distinction between those who were not involved from those who brought the disease upon themselves (Albert, 1986b). However, as the media begin to associate the disease with other groups (such as college students, children, and heterosexuals), "the stigma attached to it cannot but diminish to the degree that those who we perceive to be at significant risk belong increasingly to socially valued groups" (Albert, 1987: 39). Yet, the stigma continues to hold. Albert (1987: 39) states:

As the second largest cause of death among young adults (rapidly becoming the largest) one need only to read the obituaries of persons who die prematurely to note the ways in which its name is often avoided. Instead of AIDS, pneumonia, meningitis, or other illnesses not usually found in the young are cited as the cause of death.

Thus, obituaries provide an excellent source for illustrating the thesis of the social construction of reality through language. In the context of a stigmatized disease disproportionately affecting stigmatized groups, the language used to explain early deaths among young men reconstructs the causes in an attempt to distance the deceased person from the disease and the risk group, thereby perpetuating those very stigmas. However, as more and more people learn to decode the language, the obituaries ironically have the opposite effect of actually signaling AIDS as the real cause.

## OBITUARIES AND AIDS

For the past several years, journalists have called some attention to the dilema of reporting AIDS deaths. David Sanford (1985), in an article appearing in the August 29, 1985, issue of the *Wall Street Journal*, discusses the increase of death notices in the *New York Times* of young men in New York either not mentioning a cause or providing some telltale clue:

the death of any young man is suspect, the unmarried man particularly. If the young man is said to have died of pneumonia, lymphoma, leukemia, meningitis, or "a long illness" that he fought bravely, courageously or valiantly, the AIDS hypothesis is strengthened.

Similarly, Alexis Jetter (1986), writing in the July/August 1986 issue of the *Columbia Journalism Review*, says that many people have learned how to read between the lines by looking for the diseases most associated with AIDS as a clue. Failure to specify the cause of death as AIDS is due to the stigma of the disease as much as it is due to the person's gay identity, Jetter feels. Jetter (1986: 16) reports that "the stigma of having lost a lover or family member to AIDS may loom larger than fear of having that person exposed as a homosexual. One family threatened to sue the *Philadelphia Daily News*, not for writing an obit eulogizing their son as a prominent member of the gay community, but for saying that he died of AIDS."

Certainly, some of the language used in obituaries is a result of family members not providing the information and of the reluctance of newspapers to investigate the story with the same fervor they do other stories. But this only further illustrates the negative images associated with the disease and the groups at highest risk. By not reporting the actual cause as AIDS, the families and the euphemistic obituaries perpetuate the stigma and the sense of otherness associated with the disease and the gay subculture. Nancy Spiller, in the *Los Angeles Herald Examiner* of August 24, 1986, writes: "Despite extensive media coverage, AIDS is an invisible epidemic. The widespread public fear of acquired immune deficiency syndrome has forced many of its victims to silence. They must deny the tragic truth to their last breath because AIDS patients have become the untouchables of our age."

One of the key issues raised by obituary reporting is personal privacy versus journalistic ethics. David Shaw (1986) asks in a September 3, 1986, article in the *Los Angeles Times*, "Should a newspaper mention AIDS as a cause of death if AIDS can be proved or is openly acknowledged . . . ? Should a newspaper mention AIDS if it is only widely believed but neither acknowledged nor proved?" Unlike other diseases which often went unreported in earlier generations (such as tuberculosis or cancer), AIDS raises questions of both medical and sexual ethics. The deaths of fashion designer Perry Ellis, entertainer Liberace, and lawyer Roy Cohn brought many of these questions to the surface as newspapers and magazines had to decide whether to report AIDS as the underlying cause of death when information came either from reliable sources or rumor. The dilemmas faced by the media in these and other less famous cases draw attention to the continuing stigma attached both to the disease and to homosexuality.

In addition to questions of ethics and privacy, AIDS deaths raise the issue of state laws governing death certificates. According to an article in the February 23, 1987, issue of *Newsweek*, "Death certificates are an important AIDS information source, but their effectiveness varies from state to state, depending in part on laws governing public access to the documents" ("Counting," 1987). In California, anyone can see a death certificate, so it is estimated that approximately 17 to 20 percent of AIDS deaths go unreported as such. In New York, where death certificates are confidential and the incentive to cover up the cause of death is small, about 12 percent of AIDS deaths are concealed ("Counting," 1987). The article goes on to state that the Centers for Disease Control claim 10 percent under-reporting, primarily because most states require doctors to report AIDS deaths in confidence even if not listed on death certificates. While these explanations can account for some of the obituaries failing to mention AIDS, the point still holds: the stigma attached to the disease and to the at-risk groups results in a reconstruction of the language used to report on it in the media.

## METHODOLOGY

To illustrate this thesis, a content analysis of the trade newspaper *Variety* was conducted. *Variety* is the "bible" of the entertainment industry encompassing film, theater, television, radio, music, advertising, public relations, and allied fields. It is published in daily and weekly editions. Articles in the popular press repeatedly report the higher than usual incidence of AIDS in the entertainment fields. *Variety* also is one of a few papers that has an extensive obituary section. Most newspapers tend to report only the deaths of elites and other famous people. *Variety*'s obituaries include not only the famous, but also those known only to insiders in the business and those less known even by insiders, such as the more anonymous set builders or relatives of entertainment people. As a result, it provides a larger than normal sample of death notices than most other media.

Three years of the weekly edition of *Variety* were sampled by selecting the second issue of each month during the years 1980, 1984, and 1986. In order to get a baseline of information, 1980 was chosen since it was the last year before the first cases of AIDS were discovered. The two other selected periods represent the years before and after the news of Rock Hudson's battle with AIDS made the topic more widely discussed in the media.

For each issue, the number of obituaries for men whose age at death was listed was counted. Then, the obituaries for those men who died between the

**Table 10.1**
**18- to 50-year-old Males and Survivors Listed**

|                   | 1980        | 1984        | 1986        |
|-------------------|-------------|-------------|-------------|
| Parents/Siblings  | 9 (23.7%)   | 13 (36.1%)  | 22 (59.5%)  |
| Wife/Children     | 23 (60.5)   | 16 (44.4)   | 9 (24.3)    |
| None listed       | 6 (15.8)    | 7 (19.4)    | 6 (16.2)    |
| **TOTAL:**        | 38 (100%)   | 36 (100%)   | 37 (100%)   |

ages of 18 and 50 were coded for cause of death and who survived the deceased. Those survived only by parents and/or siblings were defined as "single" while those who were survived by a wife and/or children were considered "married." This is, of course, a rough labeling, since not all those without children and wife are necessarily single or gay. Some might have been married in the past. Similarly, not all those who are married or have children are necessarily heterosexual.

The 18-to-50-age range was chosen because the majority of AIDS deaths occur in that age group. It should also be pointed out that not all deaths among "single" men in the 18-to-50-age range attributed to cancer, pneumonia, or "long illness" are AIDS related. Furthermore, AIDS does not avoid married men, some of whom may be bisexual. Therefore, since there really is no way in knowing for sure which of the obituaries are covering up AIDS-related deaths, the figures presented here are only indirect and relative indicators of the extent of the social construction of obituaries.

What is important, however, is the overall increase between 1980, 1984, and 1986 in the percentage of death notices that report single people dying from AIDS-related diseases without specifying AIDS. The hypothesis is that as the national figures for AIDS deaths increased between 1980 and 1986, more obituaries reported cancer, pneumonia, and "lengthy illness" as causes of death among single men between the ages of 18 and 50, thereby indicating a continuing stigma attached to the disease even among a population more likely to tolerate variant life-styles.

**THE FINDINGS**

As Table 10.1 shows, there were 38 obituaries for men in the 18-to-50-age range in the twelve issues of *Variety* surveyed for the year 1980. Of these, 23 (60.5 percent) listed a wife and/or children as surviving the deceased and 9 (23.7 percent) reported only parents and/or siblings. In 1984, 16 of the 36 (44.4 percent) obituaries in the 18-to-50 age range mentioned wife and/or children, while in 1986, only 24.3 percent (9 out of 37 obituaries) did. The percentage

**Table 10.2**
**18- to 50-Year-old Males and Cause of Death Listed among "Single" Men**

|  | 1980 | 1984 | 1986 |
|---|---|---|---|
| AIDS | 0 | 1 (7.7%) | 5 (22.7%) |
| Cancer | 1 (11.1%) | 0 | 2 (9.1) |
| Lengthy Illness | 1 (11.1) | 3 (23.1) | 4 (18.2) |
| Pneumonia | 0 | 0 | 3 (13.6) |
| SUBTOTAL: | 2 (22.2) | 4 (30.8) | 14 (63.6) |
| Heart | 1 (11.1) | 2 (15.4) | 1 (4.5) |
| Other* | 6 (66.7) | 7 (53.8) | 7 (31.8) |
| Total: | 9 (100%) | 13 (100%) | 22 (100%) |

* "Other" includes accidents, suicides, and not specified. In 1986, it includes one case of meningitis and two cases of liver disease.

of obituaries listing only parents and/or siblings increased from 36.2 percent in 1984 to 59.5 percent in 1986. These results were statistically significant (chi-square = 15.566, df = 4, p<.01).

How many of these men actually died from AIDS cannot be finally determined. However, an interesting pattern emerges when analyzing the causes of death. The figures in Tables 10.2 and 10.3 present the findings. Taking just the "single" men (see Table 10.2), only one died from cancer in 1980, one from a "lengthy illness," and none from pneumonia. In 1984, 23 percent (3 out of 13) died from a "lengthy illness," none from cancer or pneumonia. However, by 1986, out of 22 deaths among the "single" 18-to-50-year-old men, two died from cancer, three from pneumonia, and four from a "lengthy illness," for a total percentage of around 41 percent, almost double from 1980 for the same three categories. This number does not even include the two deaths in 1986 from liver problems, the one case of meningitis, or the two not listing any cause of death (grouped together in "other"), all of which might be AIDS related. Furthermore, the number of obituaries that actually mentioned AIDS increased from none in 1980, one (8 percent) in 1984, and five (23 percent) in 1986.

In other words, (assuming just for the moment that all deaths due to pneumonia, cancer, and lengthy illnesses are AIDS related), the total percentage of deaths—due to these causes and to AIDS combined—among the "single" men increased from 22 percent in 1980, to 31 percent in 1984, to 64 percent in

**Table 10.3**
**18- to 50-year-old Males and Cause of Death Listed among "Married" Men**

|                | 1980       | 1984        | 1986        |
|----------------|------------|-------------|-------------|
| AIDS           | 0          | 0           | 0           |
| Cancer         | 9 (39.1%)  | 3 (18.7%)   | 1 (11.1%)   |
| Lengthy Illness| 0          | 1 (6.3)     | 0           |
| Pneumonia      | 0          | 0           | 0           |
| SUBTOTAL:      | 9 (39.1)   | 4 (25.0)    | 1 (11.1)    |
| Heart          | 4 (17.4)   | 4 (25.0)    | 3 (33.3)    |
| Other*         | 10 (43.5)  | 8 (50.0)    | 5 (55.6)    |
| Total:         | 23 (100%)  | 16 (100%)   | 9 (100%)    |

* "Other" includes accidents, suicides, and not specified.

1986. It is also interesting to note that the mean age in 1986 of those dying from pneumonia is 37.6, from lengthy illnesses is 36.7, and from AIDS is 36.1.

On the other hand, among men whose obituaries listed a wife and/or children (see Table 10.3), the percentage of deaths due to pneumonia, cancer, or a lengthy illness, decreased from nine (39 percent) in 1980, to four (25 percent) in 1984, to one (11 percent) in 1986. None had AIDS listed as a cause of death. When comparing the total number of deaths between the "singles" and "marrieds" over the three years, the results are statistically significant (chi-square = 15.13, df = 2, p<.01).

## DISCUSSION AND CONCLUSION

Although the sample size is small within each year, the data suggest an increase in the percentage of deaths due to illnesses not typically associated with men in the 18-to-50-year-old age group. Since the percentage of "single" men dying from pneumonia, cancer, or a lengthy illness is substantially greater than "married" men in 1986, and since the mean age for those who died from pneumonia and a lengthy illness is similar to those who were listed as dying from AIDS, it is reasonable to conclude that many of these are really AIDS deaths concealed in the language of more "acceptable" diseases. Furthermore, it is customary for many newspapers (and a policy of *Variety*) not to report any male lovers as survivors. When they are mentioned, they are typically referred to in the concealing language of "long-time companion." *Variety* does not even use this language; not a single case was found of any hint of a surviving male lover. Not only, then, is the stigma removed from the cause of death, but so is the stigma of an alternative gay life-style.

The decoding of obituaries also involves recognizing other phrases that reconstruct the real events. Newspapers typically use the phrase that someone died of cancer or pneumonia without attributing it to another person. However, in cases where there is a suspicion that someone did die of AIDS, newspapers often state it as follows: "his mother said he had cancer"; "a spokeswoman said he died of complications from pneumonia"; or "he died of encephalitis, said the director of [the company he founded]." All these quotations from actual obituaries appearing in the *Los Angeles Times* (April 20, 1987; August 22, 1987; February 11, 1988) indicate that the paper is not saying that the person actually died from a particular disease, only that the paper was given the information, leaving open the possibility that it could actually be from something else, such as AIDS. In each of the above cases, no indication was given that the person was married; their ages were, respectively, 49, 46, and 42 when they died; and only parents and/or siblings were listed as surviving.

Although more obituaries now include the word "AIDS" as a cause of death, this is in part due to the increasing number of people with AIDS. There is no indication, however, that the relative percentage of obituaries accurately reporting the cause of death has increased. Two recent examples typify the kinds of obituaries still appearing in newspapers. The following obituary from the *Los Angeles Times* (April 20, 1987) is a good example of the phrases used to reconstruct the stigmas: "A spokesman said he died . . . of pneumonia complicated by shigella, a parasitic disease that causes dysentery. . . . [A public relations director] said [the 39-year-old deceased man] contracted the disease during a trip." The *New York Times* (October 7, 1988) reported: "[the 57-year-old man] died of heart failure caused by a long respiratory illness, his family said. . . . He is survived by three brothers . . . and two sisters." The usual codings are there, as in *Variety*, all working to redefine the meanings and to conceal the actual stigmatizing cause of death and stigmatizing life-style. In both cases, it was later confirmed (publicly in the former case, privately in the latter) that the men had indeed contracted AIDS and were gay.

As Albert (1986a: 175–76) concluded about his own research into media reporting of AIDS, "Although media coverage of AIDS does not appear, for the most part, to have been intentionally stigmatizing, it can, in fact, be seen to have approached the story in ways that have appeared to reaffirm the outcast status of at-risk groups, especially homosexual men." Given the associations of illness, disease, and homosexuality in the public's mind, and the assumptions of personal responsibility for disease and life-style, it is not unusual to see the media (and families) act in ways which reconstruct the language used to describe an event. It's just that in the case of AIDS, it results in the unfortunate perpetuation of just those stigmas and misinformed meanings which could result in misguided social policies and fear in the general population.

## REFERENCES

Albert, Edward. 1986a. "Illness and deviance: The response of the press to AIDS, pp. 163–76. In Douglas A. Feldman and Thomas M. Johnson (eds.), *The Social Dimensions of AIDS: Method and Theory*. New York: Praeger.

———. 1986b. "Acquired immune deficiency syndrome: The victim and the press," pp. 135–58. In Thelma McCormack (ed.), *Studies in Communications*, vol. 3. Greenwich, CT: JAI Press.

———. 1987. "AIDS and the press: The creation and transformation of a social problem." Paper presented at the annual meeting of the Society for the Study of Social Problems, Chicago.

Berger, Peter, and Thomas Luckmann. 1966. *The Social Construction of Reality*. Garden City: Doubleday.

Conrad, Peter, and Joseph W. Schneider. 1980. *Deviance and Medicalization: From Badness to Sickness*. St. Louis: Mosby.

"Counting the AIDS victims." 1987. *Newsweek* (February 23): 65.

Goffman, Erving. 1963. *Stigma: Notes on the Management of a Spoiled Identity*. Englewood Cliffs, NJ: Prentice-Hall.

Jetter, Alexis. 1986. "AIDS and the obits." *Columbia Journalism Review* (July/August): 14–16.

Sanford, David. 1985. "Need we guess why young men are dying?" *Wall Street Journal* (August 29).

Shaw, David. 1986. "AIDS rumors—do they belong in news stories?" *Los Angeles Times* (September 3): 1, 18–19.

Sontag, Susan. 1978. *Illness as Metaphor*. New York: Farrar, Straus and Giroux.

Spiller, Nancy. 1986. "AIDS: Portraits of 20 People." *Los Angeles Herald Examiner* (August 24): E–1, E–10.

# Chapter Eleven

## Sex, Politics, and Guilt: A Study of Homophobia and the AIDS Phenomenon

### Norris G. Lang

This chapter examines the contribution made by homophobia, as a psychological complex, to the disease of AIDS as a cultural phenomenon. More precisely, it lays out the manner in which two system-maintaining ideologies—"blaming the victim" and "sham"—direct the path homophobia takes in the presence of AIDS. The focus of the discussion is on the individual, the gay male with AIDS, and on his choice for dealing with the onset of his disease in terms of the maintenance or creation of social relationships. The assumption taken by the author of this chapter is that homophobia, as it is internalized by the person with AIDS (PWA), affects the very interaction in which he engages.

It is as if there exists a continuum, measuring greater and lesser degrees of social activity, along which a PWA positions himself. At one end of this continuum is a PWA who is heavily secretive and isolated, in gay parlance— "in the closet." A social leper, a psychological pariah, he wears his mantle of "normalcy" like a disguise to protect himself from the psychological and social rejection he expects from others. At the other end of this hypothetical continuum, a heuristic device in the best Redfieldian tradition (Redfield 1962:232), is a PWA who has not only successfully learned to reach out to others but also to involve himself continuously in the creation of social ties. For more recently reported PWAs who survive longer than the typical 18 months after diagnosis, this ability for continually creating social ties protects him from the isolation that would result from the "burnout" often alluded to by friends and lovers who cannot sustain a social tie with someone who has a catastrophic illness and who survives longer than expected.

The points made in this chapter are derived from an ongoing study of the psychological and sociological impact of AIDS on the community of Montrose, the principal gay neighborhood of Houston, Texas. The observations described are based on interviews with over 200 gay males made between 1983 and 1988 during the course of this fieldwork. While many of the comments may appear to be based on impressionistic notions, they are grounded in several years of ethnography. This chapter is not the product of a controlled experiment that measures the covariation of certain variables, but rather is a by-product, an epiphenemenon, of doing fieldwork in this community.

Yet, this study is also a personal document, a kind of intellectual autobiography. Much of the nuance in this chapter is based on the author's cultural and psychological self. As Nancy Scheper-Hughes (1987:450) so sensitively and accurately tells us, writing about interaction between the anthropologist and his or her informants, cultural understanding is essentially produced, not merely recovered. She continues:

We no longer try to approach the world . . . as a fixed array of objects, but rather as a reality that cannot be fully separated from our perceptions of it. It shifts over time and in response to our gaze. It interacts with us. And the knowledge that it yields must always be interpreted by us, by the particular kind of complex social, cultural and psychological self that we bring with us into the field. This "self" cannot be denied. It structures the questions we ask and filters what we see and hear as well as what we do not think to ask or fail to see and hear.

The majority of the larger population of respondents are members of that category known as the "worried well." These gay men are individuals who are concerned about their membership in a group whose sexual behaviors are considered "at-risk," but have not been tested for HIV and do not exhibit any of the symptoms associated with having an immune system that is compromised. Others fall into the remaining categories of the biomedical model of AIDS: seronegative (those who test negative for the human immunodeficiency virus), seropositive (those who test positive for the virus), persons with AIDS-related complex (PWARCs), and PWAs. PWARCs are individuals who test positive for the human immunodeficiency virus (HIV), whose immune systems are compromised, but who do not have a diagnosed opportunistic infection or AIDS-related cancer that would identify them as a PWA.

The analysis has benefited from perceptions supplied by various humanistic, anthropological frameworks. A particularly useful one has been the interactionist and labeling perspective, referred to by Berger and Luckmann (1966) as the "social construction of reality" approach. Ethnographic observations as well as reflections upon them by the author have convinced him of the necessity of adding a neo-Freudian focus. The past, as well as the present, is taken into account for a fuller analysis.

The goal of this chapter, then, is to explore the changes experienced by a gay male in his social relationships and the extent and manner in which these changes have affected his mental health. In this context, "mental health" refers to an individual's ability to create, engage in, and maintain important social relationships beyond the need for sexual gratification. As the study progressed, it became more apparent to the author that the outcome of events occurring in the present have been set in motion long ago in an individual's life history. The patterns of behavior established during an individual's formative years, especially his learned responses to a crisis situation, condition to a considerable extent his future response to a life-threatening illness such as AIDS.

AIDS has considerable influence in producing changes in an individual's network of social relationships. As AIDS has been bandied about with the labels "gay plague" or "gay cancer," its diagnosis can awaken dormant, or exacerbate active, feelings and attitudes of homophobia. Guilt is everywhere an initial emotional response. The important point, however, is that different individuals have learned different ways of processing the guilt. But in each case, the response appears to conform to the traditional, patterned way of handling stigma for that particular individual.

These techniques for managing stigma do not merely represent a set of responses stemming from AIDS as a disease phenomenon (which could be singled out and labeled as disease-phobia or AIDS-phobia). "Blaming the victim" and "sham," two system-maintaining ideologies, frame social relationships in the face of AIDS. The former is an example of the social construction of reality approach; the latter is more closely associated with a neo-Freudian perspective. In passages below, the role that "sham" plays in the socialization patterns is described, and the contribution provided by "blaming the victim" is detailed. Each system-maintaining ideology provides us with a partial blueprint for networking social ties employed by gay men. Together they present a more complete accounting of the maintenance and creation of social ties, especially by PWAs.

These ideologies, simultaneously considered, permit reflections upon the *varied* responses by gay men to AIDS as a cultural phenomenon. Homophobia, as it masks itself in these ideologies, can be accounted for from recent and current interaction as well as from a much earlier period in an individual's life history.

## HOMOPHOBIA

Let us begin with a discussion of homophobia generally, and then move on to a consideration of these system-maintaining ideologies. The goal is to pinpoint more precisely the contribution each makes to the presentation of social relationships in the face of AIDS. Homophobia refers to the fear by heterosexuals (and by some gays) of being in close quarters with homosexuals; among gays themselves, it refers to self-loathing.

Homophobia also is a general cultural phenomenon that has been used to explain two different pathologies. On the one hand, it has been used to explain a cultural pathology among "straights" (i.e., heterosexuals), and, on the other, it has been used by psychological observers, analysts, and clinicians as an explanation for a particular pathology among gays. Since homophobia invariably affects the lives of gay men, the expression of homophobic attitudes is well known to them.

Although as a psychological concept it refers to the fear of same sex, in the present context, the author further identifies it as a process of internalization. Every male, gay or straight, after all, has been raised in a household with parents who participate in a heterosexual relationship; in his socialization, he has been liberally exposed, we may assume, to their biases and values. Among these are those associated with sexual orientation. The dominant society's values and attitudes toward homosexuals and homosexuality, along with other attitudes transmitted during socialization, then, are internalized or introjected.

The system-maintaining ideologies mentioned above channel those biases associated with the socialization of homophobic attitudes in particular ways that involve them with certain repressive economic and political behaviors that in the popular media have come to be associated with AIDS. When the source for attitudes of homophobia is external, at the group level, the system-maintaining ideology that malfunctions from the point of view of gay males is "blaming the victim" (Crawford 1977; Margolis 1982; Riessman 1983; Ryan 1976). The operation of this ideology allows for the inequity of sexual gender and orientation as a pervasive characteristic for major portions of American society to remain unchecked.

When the origin for the attitudes of homophobia is internally derived, at the individual level, the system-maintaining ideology is "sham," the preference for the production of a counterfeit society over one that recognizes the diversity in needs and behaviors of all its citizens. Only gradually does each gay male in his growing-up years become aware, with respect to his sexual orientation, of his being different, of his separateness, from members of his own family and other social groupings. "Sham" permits this individual to play out a charade of conformity as a process of managing his stigma (Goffman 1963). The gay male child or adolescent is allowed to save face by pretending to be that which he is not—a heterosexual. In those instances where he does not exhibit the appropriate behavior, a sense of personal shame can be imposed by members from these groups in an effort to bring his outward behavior more into alignment with the expected internal norm.

## HOMOPHOBIA AND SYSTEM-MAINTAINING IDEOLOGIES

In this section, the author wishes to pinpoint the ways in which these system-maintaining ideologies articulate with homophobic attitudes, both among heterosexuals and among gays. Homophobia then prepares the way in which AIDS as a cultural phenomenon becomes embedded. According to Margolis (1982:213), the creation of ideologies that perpetuate the status quo represents malfunctions in a culture's social and economic structure. The need for these ideologies, she continues, is greater in those societies that are stratified into haves and have-nots and whose resulting tension represents a challenge to the established order. In applying this view of social inequality and inequity to the gay community, an important contrast with other stigmatized minorities is sharply brought into focus.

The discrimination against gays is not always primarily or directly economic. As a consequence of their chameleonlike status, many men can shed or take on a public gay identity at will depending on the appropriateness of the particular context. The phenomenon of "passing," a process more in tune with white expectations for black behavior of two generations ago, is an ability gays possess that is extraordinarily pervasive.

Discrimination against gays in Houston is primarily political and reflects the growing recognition, or at least perception, of their greater political influence as a result of increased internal unity (Lang 1987). The forces bringing about extensive internal political solidarity are the same forces that are responsible for the transformation of gay men from the label of sexual "perverts" or "deviants" to their inclusion into a minority group, a subculture. The media attention surrounding AIDS has added immeasurably to this political visibility. In their quest to sensationalize the AIDS phenomena, the media has expanded its forum for both progay and antigay forces to bring their respective points of view to the public. The agenda for this forum extends beyond AIDS and includes the political presence of gays in the Houston area.

### "Blaming the Victim"

Ryan (1976:10) declares that "blaming the victim" depends on a process of identification " . . . whereby the victim . . . is identified as strange, different—in other words, as a barbarian, a savage." He (1976:10–11) continues that this is how the distressed and disinherited are redefined in order to make it possible for us to look at society's problems and to attribute their causation to the individuals affected. Aspiring "victim" blamers are compelled to stress that " 'these people' think in different forms, act in different patterns, cling to different truths." But what they do not emphasize is that this is yet another technique for social manipulation, a means of portraying social ills in ways that favor the status quo.

As Margolis (1982:213) declares in her discussion of ideology and sexual discrimination in the contemporary United States, "blaming the victim" helps to cover up the liability of the conditions of inequality and discrimination under which that group lives. With respect to the situation involving gay males in Houston, misrepresentation of facts was widely used as demogoguery in the campaign for a gay rights ordinance (Lang 1987), a factor conforming to Ryan's original introduction (referred to in Margolis 1982:213) where he recognized that "blaming the victim" consists, wherever and whenever it occurs, of a set of officially certified non-facts.

### "Sham"

In his book, *Pathways to Madness*, Jules Henry (1973:99) informs us that "sham" is a combination of concealment and pretense. We conceal that which we really feel and we pretend we feel something different. He goes on to point out that this capacity for "sham" is truly universal and, as a consequence, is a part of human nature. He writes that social life and good manners compel deception for even the most truly innocent and well-intentioned among us. "Engineered by fear, sham is a bridge between the undesirable and the necessary, making the undesirable useful and the necessary bearable." He continues, "The real problem is not whether to be a sham, but to understand when to drop the mask and when to put it on" (1973:99).

Goffman (1963:130) makes the point that stigma management is a general feature of society, a process that occurs wherever there are identity norms. In his more general usage, the present author sees his concept of stigma management as comparable to what Jules Henry discusses as "sham." Bock (1988:150), commenting on Goffman's work on stigma, writes that, since we are all stigmatized relative to some category of "normals," guilt lies at the basis of all social organization. So while Goffman's concept might lead us to this conclusion, as it did for Bock, Henry's concept of "sham" might lead us to reason that deceit or passing, conforming to the identity norms, lies at the basis of all social organization.

Jules Henry likens social life to a set of concentric circles ranging from the ideal circle of "truth" located innermost to the circle of "sham" located outermost. At each movement outward, the obligation to be open about our feelings diminishes and the obligation to conceal increases. In this model, concealment becomes an ever more important social obligation as we move outwardly from our closest relationships to others that are significantly less so. When his concentric-circle model of social life is reversed, he asserts we have pathology. If "truth" is expected in the outerworld and "sham" in the family, according to Henry, then, we have a pathological situation that he defines as a pathway to madness.

It is Henry's (1973:100) description of mental pathology that projects the gay males' process of socialization into stark relief. His pathological pathway is standard fare for young, closeted homosexuals in straight communities across the American landscape. As we shall observe later, the individual's broader dealings and attitudes concerning his sexual orientation determine whether this reversal leads to pathology or merely to a strategy for coping. Those who work this situation out as a strategy for coping are in truth masters of, in Henry's terms, the essence of being middle class (referring to the ability to get along in life without too much misery by being able at every moment to manage "sham").

## HOMOPHOBIA AND ITS IDEOLOGIES

As homophobia in American society appears to be a common phenomenon, it lends itself most significantly to the creation of the ghetto-like status of gay neighborhoods. And in this respect, it has a direct role in setting the stage for AIDS. Gays as a subcultural grouping are marked off from the larger society by virtue of their sexual orientation. As a consequence of this situation, sexually oriented businesses catering to gay social activities—gay baths, bookstores, leather boutiques, and pornographic theaters—are concentrated in these areas of the city offering gay men easy access to frequent, anonymous, and impersonal sex, often times next door or down the street.

Until recently, the bars and other establishments offering entertainment glorified the "fast-lane" fantasies so often considered by many outsiders to be synonymous with the gay life-style. Youth, sex, some drugs, parties, leather, and, to a lesser extent, sado-masochistic practices were held up to the gay male as valued and worthy of being sought after. Publications, posters, and signs paid ample testimony to the superior status of this fast-lane, multiple-partnered, anonymous sexual life-style as the normal way of living gay, a way touted for its atypically non-Western, unabashed devotion to pleasure. Gays are self-righteously acclaimed for having broken the shackles of the puritanical, heterosexual life-style where sexual desire is met with "measured denial" (White 1983:68).

The point is that the prevalency of this attitude derives from the nearly universal presence of homophobia in this culture. Some gays accept this self-indulgent presentation of life; others do not. Those who do represent the group most seriously at-risk for contracting AIDS. In this respect, Montrose in Houston is comparable to Harlem in the 1920s when blacks from all walks of life and from all economic strata lived in the same neighborhood. Much of the internal political machinations within Montrose, for example, represent attempts on the part of the more affluent to distance themselves in publicity and in geography from the "street people."

For the moment, let us consider this situation from the standpoint of "sham." Gay male youths spend their childhoods among straights learning the correctness of social skills enabling them to hide their identities as homosexuals. Many such youths experience the culture's rituals of courtship, dating, and even mating with clammy hands, feigned excitement, counterfeit enthusiasm, and concealed anxiety. They play out the sham of heterosexual behavior, thereby hoping to allay any suspicions about their true desires.

And true to the structure of "gay sham," while they conceal the most important truths about themselves from those most closely related to them, they engage in activities of the most intimate kind with the males they met only moments before and many times will never see again. These individuals, then, have learned a successful strategy of "sham"; they eventually come to compartmentalize their lives into public and personal, to not allow these two facets of their lives to be intertwined any more than is absolutely necessary. Concealment becomes a self-protecting strategy. Their homophobia directs them to deny their homosexuality while interacting in the straight world. They project the discrimination they fear would otherwise ensue.

The situation which drew my interest to this problem came from comments made by various alternative health care providers in the course of our ongoing study of the sociological and psychological correlates of AIDS in the gay community of Houston, Texas (see Kotarba and Lang 1986; Lang and Kotarba 1984). One, a physical therapist and masseur, who said that he had worked with over 60 AIDS patients, related that his typical patient was a loner, a person who previously lived and organized his entire social life around cruising (i.e., looking for and possibly meeting a sexual partner) and the casual sexual encounter. Another alternative health care provider, whose role as a peer counselor qualifies him to help the person with AIDS accept his disease, described his biggest problem as being one of helping many of these individuals develop the simplest of social skills. In other words, some of his clients, before contracting this disease, were incapable of any meaningful social relationship other than one which is sexual. Or, as Edmund White (1983) described it, in his article on "Sexual Culture," such men compress the entire life cycle into the space of the "one night stand."

For these individuals, then, it appears as if sex becomes an organizing theme for their cultural experience. But while some of these individuals might be described as "compulsively addicted" to sex, they compromise only one segment of the gay community. Others among them are sexually active with multiple-partnered sex; but this sexual activity takes place under a sense of personal control and from a rationally based desire. There are substantial numbers of still others for whom sex is but one entry among many on the social menu. AIDS has touched, influenced, and marked them all.

## PRE-AIDS: GAY LIBERATION AND THE GHETTO (1969–81)

### The Emergence of "Swish" Heights

During the 1960s and earlier, society, judges, religious leaders, doctors, teachers, and parents, not homosexuality, provided the gay person with a mental and behavioral pathology. He was not actually sick (we now know), but society created a sick role for him. And unfortunately, all too often, the gay individual having nowhere to turn for affirmation acquiesced in this sickness diagnosis. Homosexuals are still viewed as sinful, criminal, or deviant by members of the dominant society. Whether they favor a religious, legal, or medical diagnosis, a gay person is looked on as less than "normal," as handicapped, at best "perverted" and at worst dangerous.

Between 1969 and 1981, the gay liberation social movement fostered a new view of the homosexual, one crafted by gays themselves. This new identity or role allows for self-actualization without negative overtones. As a group, gays involved themselves in the construction of this new social identity and, with the new image and life-styles associated with it, emerged during the 1970s as a new minority, a subculture. Gays no longer predominantly acted as isolated individuals in one-to-one relationships, for example doctor-patient, with the larger, heterosexual society. Now they were provided with the ability to deal with the larger society as a member of a minority group (Lang and Kotarba 1984).

Research on gays also shifted during this same period, from a concern on the part of medical practitioners with the etiology of homosexuality, the cause or causes for this medical pathology, to more social, cultural, and political analyses of their behavior, for example D'Emilio (1983:238–39). Like the blacks and Hispanic-Americans before them, they had arrived. They developed their own tastes and attitudes, their own heroes, their own codes of proper behavior. Now they could move into their own ghettos, eat at their own restaurants, drink in their own bars, and attend movies in their own theaters. They could promote their own sources for diversion, such as gay baths and gay bookstores. They adopted their own styles for dress, published their own newspapers, magazines, and books, worshiped in their own churches and synagogues, and opened their own shops, services, and businesses. They worked out in their own gyms and, in some cases, provided their own security patrols. They even have their own specialized chapters of Alcoholics Anonymous and Overeaters Anonymous.

They came more and more to identify with one another and to develop positive feelings for their own identity. At last, they had become a suitable topic for the social scientist. Anthropologists, sociologists, ethnolinguists, political scientists, and even historians could now freely undertake studies of people who engage in same sex conduct without necessarily sullying their own reputation.[1]

## THE ERA OF AIDS: 1981 UNTIL THE PRESENT

The ghetto provides the gay male with an inconsistent situation. As Edmund White (1983:68) writes, "The very universality of sexual opportunity within the modern gay ghetto has, paradoxically, increased the importance of friendship." While Mr. White is drawing attention to the same inconsistency that I am, he does it in a more positive light. The gay ghetto, like a two-edged sword, cuts in two ways. As White states, it does increase the importance of friendship, yet it also presents a situation that mushrooms the incidence of sexually transmitted diseases (STDs). The pre-AIDS situation allowed many observers of the gay scene to treat the incidence of STDs as something that should be displayed, like merit badges for an Eagle scout.

These discussions, however, do not take into account the sobering presence of AIDS. As one informant described changes in his way of thinking about the subject of sexual freedom:

I have had some thought about my community and the problems we have relating one with another. It has caused me to do some thinking. For instance, the fact that gay men tend to have sex with strangers and not their friends. This does not apply to lesbians. A lesbian one night stand takes three weeks. Once you become somebody's good friend ... if you start off sexually, you become lovers or you become good friends, at which point you have excluded that person, because now you're friends. I think this is unfortunate because this leads to existential loneliness. The bond between men is . . . I don't think it's whole. I don't think it's put together properly. I think love or friendship is a caring sexual encounter and we don't do that. We save that kind of intimacy for people we don't know.

This gay male is still not ready to totally abandon his rejection of the heterosexual life-style, however. He continues,

The older I get the more awareness is coming in. I have been thinking about this in terms of my own self. In terms of the way I relate to other people, other gay men. I don't relate to straight people at all. We have been talking among some of us about starting some sort of club where we have, or agree, to be sexually active within that group only and to practice safe sex.

Gays prior to 1981 were basking in the light of their newfound freedoms. Society seemed not so incongenial after all. Then came the Moral Majority and Reaganomics. The gay political problem and the "gay plague" both seemed to be fortuitous scapegoats. For the leaders of these conservatives, AIDS presented a just and deserved specter, one riddled with "God's judgment" on this "heinous" life-style. They appear compelled to continue their unabated repression and recrimination of gays. AIDS either exacerbates this situation or is used as a vehicle to augment discrimination. They rally around the flag of divisiveness and bigotry. They employ "gay baiting" to win local political contests. They unashamedly make use of demogoguery in their efforts to gain political control (Lang 1987). The two system-maintaining ideologies—"blaming the victim" and "sham"—are utilized most effectively in their campaign for political control. AIDS has been politicized beyond the wildest fears of the leaders of the Lesbian and Gay Political Caucus in Houston and other community leaders by these conservatives to wrest control away from more moderate factions in Houston's political arena.

Since the early 1980s, gay leaders who have emerged in response to AIDS have taken a different tack. Now, the life-style in and of itself is not evil, bad, or wrong. However, until a cure or a method of prevention is discovered, gays are told to curb the most extreme acts associated with their sexuality, to practice "safe-sex," to turn toward a more monogamous, coupled way of living gay. Courtship and romance are trendy behaviors representing positive affirmation of this new and restrained way of living sexually.

The social psychology of these historically derived sets of circumstances established two poles between which a gay male could, or could not, come to terms with his own homosexuality. My ethnographic experiences thus far lead me to believe that an individual's degree of closetedness is the single most important variable in determining whether his overall response to the AIDS phenomenon will be life supporting or life threatening; whether that individual will morbidly preoccupy himself with his death and allow the extinction of his life to become the cornerstone of his remaining days or whether he will celebrate his experience as a part of his total life. Both "coming out" and an individual's acceptance of AIDS are processes, not determinate points of reference in an individual's life history.

Preliminary impressions indicate some other variables related to the PWA's response to his disease are the age of the informant, the amount or intensity of support he receives from family and friends, the degree to which his daily life is pain-free, whether or not his "coming-out" occurred prior to the gay liberation movement or afterwards, and his degree of personal familiarity with the AIDS phenomenon. In turn, these variables affirm the degree to which an individual compartmentalized his life into discrete social spheres as a practical defense mechanism, an example of Goffman's (1963:130) process of stigma management. His acceptance, positively or negatively, of his own homosexuality is mirrored in the degree to which he maintains an integration of these social spheres—private and public, career and sexual, or others.

There are individuals who keep sexual relationships totally apart from public and private networks of social relationships. There are other individuals, for whom sex tends always to be anonymous, whose social and occupational lives may or may not be sharply segregated. And there are still other individuals who successfully integrate the private, public, and sexual spheres of their lives.

When there exists a high degree of overlap of representatives from these various groups, the individual more than likely will deal with the AIDS phenomenon in a nearly guilt-free, sham-free manner. Actually, it is not that he is "sham-free" as much as it is that he has learned to manage "sham" without pathology.

The more sharply segregated these social spheres of life, the more highly fractionated his life is into these diverse spheres, the more compartmentalized his social life, and the more self-recrimination that the individual experiences, the nearer to the pole for pathological "sham" and negative self-evaluation he lies. In Goffman's (1963:123) framework, his management of stigma has encouraged him to accept for himself a self that is "a resident alien, a voice of the group that speaks for him and through him."

Those gay men who are "out of the closet," living an active gay life in Montrose, must be distinguished from those gay men who remain "in the closet." Those who remain in the closet, made sick and provided a mental pathology as a result of the sham devised by history, society, and their personal life histories, are the least prepared to deal with AIDS either as a disease or as a cultural phenomenon.

They take their sex like a thief in the night. Their fractionated lives spell their fate and seal their doom. Several "closeted" individuals have asked their doctors not to diagnose and report their condition. These men do not avail themselves of the support groups that are available, the group therapy, the peer counseling, the special knowledge that has been gleaned from the care and research of previous AIDS patients to make their remaining days a little more bearable, a little less pain-ridden, isolated and alone. They will die as they lived, their lives a total sham. No one socially significant to them other than themselves will ever know the most important truths about their lives, and, now, their deaths. They cloak their death in half-truths, secrecy, and mystery to the same degree that previously they seized their sex.

Many gays have been forced to deny their sexuality and sexual orientation for many years. No matter what the pace of the life-style that is eventually assumed by a gay male, almost invariably upon arriving in a gay ghetto, a period of unlicensed sexual revelry ensues, at a level that most heterosexual men could only fantasize. Eventually, however, this life-style sates the appetites of its adherents, and other factors come into play, many of them also related to homophobia, that channel some gays into a conservative life-style, but others into the maintenance of this "fast-lane" life-style.

The flamboyancy of this life-style, its eroticism, its overwhelming dedication to excess is a direct outcome of the larger society's negative attitudes toward same-sex conduct, and an example of "blaming the victim." Whether due to biology or culture, males in this society are encouraged to think about and deal with their sexuality in a more open and polypartnering way than are females (Feldman 1988). Add drugs and alcohol to this mixture and you have a lively combination for promoting this fast-paced life-style. Gay males cocooned in their ghettos, having learned "sham" and concealment as a strategy for surviving (as a process for managing stigma), much more so than their "straight" counterparts, are encouraged to live out their most extreme fantasies. Were it not for gay liberation, this side of gay life would amount to no more than a caricature for being gay and possibly be more typical, accurate and uniform. This social construction of gay reality, as Goffman (1963:123) writing about the special situation of the stigmatized has said, is derived from society because "before a difference can matter much it must be conceptualized collectively by the society as a whole."

However, gay liberation and the ensuing minoritization of gays allow a situation to unfold where at last gays have come to the possibility and the realization that there can be many ways of living gay. Many individuals now can develop, more often than previously, the kinds of permanent, stable, long-term relationships once thought possible only within the cloistered domain of heterosexuality. Low self-esteem and lack of options are more conducive to creating and maintaining this at-risk life-style than is "male nature" or homosexuality itself. In fact, for many men living active gay lives in Montrose, homophobia takes its toll in low self-esteem, alcoholism, drug addiction, sexual addiction, and other compulsive behaviors.

## CONCLUSION

AIDS is a medical condition which among gay men has grown to epidemic proportions and threatens to grow significantly further. Homophobia is expressed in all quarters; from the person with AIDS in the form of guilt and shame, from his family and friends in the form of rejection, from the gay community at large in the form of denial and apathy, from the medical profession in the form of ignorance, and from the dominant heterosexual society in the form of benign neglect.

Many heterosexuals still regard the homosexual as "perverted." As if they were caught in a time warp from the 1950s, they proclaim that AIDS is God's punishment for the arrogance, the sin, and the moral heresy of the gay militant. AIDS as a medical pathology has placed homosexuality to an even greater extent in a negative ambience and the homosexual even more so in the role of cultural pariah, molester of children, and vile recruiter of adolescents. This social construction of gay reality promotes "blaming the victim" and "sham" too very often as the method of control and division from within.

## NOTE

An earlier version of this chapter was read at the annual meetings of the Southwestern Social Science Association in March 1985. Acknowledgement and appreciation are given to Evelyn A. Early and Kenneth L. Brown, University of Houston, and George L. Hicks, Brown University, for having commented on this earlier draft. Financial support for the fieldwork was provided by a seed grant from the Center for Public Policy, College of Social Sciences, University of Houston.

1. For example, Jules Henry (1963:265), in his book *Culture Against Man*, felt it necessary to include a footnote at the bottom of the page 265 pointing out that, "The Researcher is an unusually handsome youth with an 'adequate masculine record.' " In the narrative provided in the text, the research assistant was explaining his statement that he did not have the "nerve to dance with any of those girls." For some reason Henry felt that an explanation for this comment was necessary and as a consequence, he underscored the rationale that the reluctance to dance with these "girls" was not based on his fear of them, but that it was based on the researcher's ignorance of the dance steps and not from his sexual orientation.

## REFERENCES

Bock, Philip K. 1988. Rethinking Psychological Anthropology, Continuity and Change in the Study of Human Action.

Crawford, Robert. 1977. You are Dangerous to your Health: The Idealogy and Politics of Victim Blaming. In *International Journal of Health Services*, volume 7, number 4.

D'Emilio, John. 1983. *Sexual Politics, Sexual Communities: The Making of a Homosexual Minority in the United States*. Chicago: The University of Chicago Press.

Feldman, Douglas A. 1988. Personal communication.

Goffman, Erving. 1963. *Stigma, Notes on the Management of Spoiled Identity*. Englewood Cliffs, NJ: Prentice-Hall.

Henry, Jules. 1973. *Pathways to Madness*. New York: Vintage Books.

———. 1963. *Culture Against Man*. New York: Random House.

Kotarba, Joseph A., and Norris G. Lang. 1986. Gay Lifestyle Change Since AIDS as Preventive Health Care. In Douglas A. Feldman and Thomas Johnson, (eds.), *The Social Dimensions of AIDS: Method and Theory*, pp. 127–43. New York: Praeger.

Lang, Norris G. 1987. Gays, AIDS, and the Ballot Box: The Politics of Disease. In *Medical Anthropology*. In press.

Lang, Norris G., and Joseph A. Kotarba. 1984. The Remedicalization of Homosexuality Since AIDS. Unpublished ms.

Margolis, Maxine. 1982. Blaming the Victim: Ideology and Sexual Discrimination in the Contemporary United States. In Conrad Phillip Kottak, (ed.), *Researching American Culture: A Guide for Student Anthropologists*, pp. 212–26. Ann Arbor: University of Michigan Press.

Redfield, Robert. 1962. The Folk Society. In Margaret Park Redfield, (ed.), *Human Nature and the Study of Society: The Papers of Robert Redfield, Volume 1*, pp. 231–53. Chicago: The University of Chicago Press.

Riessman, Catherine Kohler. 1983. Women and Medicalization: A New Perspective. *Social Policy*, volume 14, Summer, pp. 3–18.

Ryan, William. 1976. *Blaming the Victim*. New York: Vintage Books.

Scheper-Hughes, Nancy. 1987. The Margaret Mead Controversy: Culture, Biology and Anthropological Inquiry. In Herbert Applebaum, (ed.), *Perspectives in Cultural Anthropology*, pp. 443–54. Albany: State University of New York Press.

White, Edmund. 1983. Sexual Culture. *Vanity Fair*. December, 64–68.

# Chapter Twelve

## Increasing the Cost of Living: Class and Exploitation in the Delivery of Social Services to Persons with AIDS

### Juliet A. Niehaus

In the human service professions, social services are traditionally cast as the products and activities of the formally organized government or voluntary agencies which function to ameliorate social problems and promote communal well-being (Weissman 1983:186). Social services include monetary assistance, in-kind aid such as free meals, clothing or housing,[1] and what are often termed "soft services." This final category includes supportive services such as counseling and educational programs. Although the term "social services" primarily refers to governmental or nonprofit assistance, in capitalist economies private sector profit-making agencies may also provide many of these services either independently or under government contracts. Furthermore, inadequacy or unavailability of formal-level services can, as Stack (1974) for example has shown, result in the elaboration of "informal" modes of social assistance such as that provided by family and friend support networks.[2]

Since the onset of the AIDS epidemic in the early 1980s, services on all three levels—governmental/voluntary, private profit-making, and informal—have emerged to respond to the complex needs of those who have become ill with the disease. Federal, state, and local programs have aimed to consolidate and prioritize monetary assistance and general support services for persons with AIDS (PWAs). Voluntary nonprofit organizations have developed counseling services, buddy programs, and meal delivery services, and offer legal and financial advocacy and educational information. In the private profit sector, medical home care agencies provide skilled nursing care, intravenous drug infusion supplies and services, and specially trained home health aides to tend to the personal care needs of the ill PWA. When necessary, informal support networks of family and friends supplement, or even at times replace, formal organizations in the provision of both economic and social assistance.

This chapter examines the assistance available to PWAs in New York City and discusses class variation in the experience of AIDS as this is revealed through use of private, formal, and informal levels of assistance. The importance of class to an understanding of the AIDS experience has been only peripherally addressed. Emphasis has been primarily placed on "risk group" (i.e., gay men, intravenous drug users (IVDUs), transfusion recipients, heterosexual partners of IVDUs) as the major variable in the psychosocial problems faced throughout the illness.[3] The risk group is not necessarily a cultural entity, however. The notion of "risk group" emerges from the scientific community's focus on the biology of transmission. In some cases, risk groups may have cultural characteristics.[4] In all cases, risk groups are cross-cut by class, regional, religious, and ethnic differentials which render the risk group category an only partially meaningful measure of the illness experience. Focus on the risk group then as a unit of study can obscure our understanding of the influence of other potent sociocultural groupings on both the course and costs of the illness. This chapter's portrayal of the way in which class contributes to varied experiences of AIDS within one particular risk group demonstrates this, and points toward the deeper understanding of AIDS in the United States which we can gain from more culturally aware analyses.

The experiences discussed are those of gay and bisexual men in New York City. Their ages range from 30 to 50, with most in their late thirties or early forties.[5] Research material was derived from two sources of equal importance. First, consistent with traditional anthropological methodology, open-ended interviews were conducted with PWAs and with social workers, nurses, doctors, and home care personnel who work with them. Second, since many of the PWAs discussed were at some point patients at New York University Medical Center where the author holds a position as social worker, there is considerable reliance on material gathered through participant observation of PWAs both during and after hospitalization.

The medical social work role includes both counseling and discharge planning. The latter involves evaluation of the PWA's post-hospital needs, both medical and psychosocial, and ensuring that these are provided for at discharge. Such planning brings with it direct knowledge of availability of services, insurance coverage dilemmas, and of the intersection of such issues with the PWA's support network. As discharge planner, one becomes aware of the PWA's needs and resources on all levels—economic, social, and psychological—and of his ability to fulfill his desires in relation to his available resources. As counselor, one enters the actual process of decision making around care, and observes firsthand the conflicts, struggles, and nuances of this process. I witnessed not only the successful outcome of decision making, but the pain, anger, and frustration that attended lapses in insurance or failures in support systems. I likewise shared in the excruciating difficulties surrounding whether to accept or reject forms of care or treatment which might merely prolong a PWA's suffering. Much of what is presented here is in tribute to the courage of these PWAs in their efforts to live with the outcome of their disease with dignity. Much is also offered as an indictment of their agonies.

The material presented reflects an eighteen month period from June 1987 through November 1988 during which work was done with over 50 PWAs. The group was predominantly what the Ehrenreichs (1979) term "professional-managerial class." "Class" in their usage does not refer to income level, but to an historically defined position in the structure of economic relationships within the society (ibid.:10). This professional-managerial class comprises " . . . salaried mental workers who do not own the means of production and whose major function in the social division of labor may be described broadly as the *reproduction* of capitalist culture and capitalist class relations" (ibid.:12). Occupations and skills are wide-ranging. Specifically, this class would include professionals involved in the reproduction of social belief systems and knowledge (e.g., teachers, social workers, psychologists, entertainers, advertising and media professionals). It would also include middle-level administrators and managers, engineers, and technical workers who are the actual implementors of the corporations, foundations, and other institutions owned by the capitalist class. The Ehrenreichs also argue that certain cultural features, specifically family structure, patterns of marriage and child rearing and the value placed on education characterize professional-managerial class membership (ibid.:29–30, 325).

The professionals with AIDS upon whom this work is based do exhibit many similarities in the objective conditions of life affecting the disease experience. Most are covered by corporate group plan health insurance policies which provide extensive benefits, especially for home care, resulting in significant commonalities of experience regarding options for post-hospital care. Family and social network members have similar occupational life-styles, educational levels, and family values which impact on the course of illness. Overall the experience of AIDS appears very different for these professionals than for those less affluent PWAs for whom economic need results in major tensions around basic subsistence, housing, and medical care, and in struggles with public welfare bureaucracies.[6] It is arguable though whether dying of AIDS, or living with it, is any easier for the more affluent. Where AIDS is concerned, resources can certainly engender more potential for choices around treatment and care. Yet such options carry with them a separate set of dilemmas in modern society. And while economic costs may be less of an issue, as will be shown here, the emotional and social costs of the care options offered can be vast.

## FORMAL SERVICES AND THE PROFESSIONAL WITH AIDS

Formal responses to the social service needs of PWAs include: 1) government provisions through the traditional public assistance and welfare structures;

2) government provisions through public health department programming; and
3) services and programs offered by voluntary nonprofit organizations.

### Public Assistance and Welfare Programs

Most governmental assistance for PWAs has been channelled through already existing welfare and health care system structures. The PWA's access to federal, state, and local programs is contingent upon fulfilling eligibility requirements. As with most government public assistance programs, services for PWAs are primarily aimed at those who are economically needy or who have been rendered destitute because of the disease. For only one program, Social Security Disability (SSD), is income not the major criterion for eligibility. PWAs can receive SSD payments so long as they have not collected wages for five months and have worked the required period of time.[7] The Medicare hospitalization insurance that accompanies Social Security payments for the elderly does not, however, automatically come to those receiving SSD. There is a two-year waiting period for this benefit which makes Medicare coverage essentially out of the question for most PWAs whose life span following establishment of disability rarely passes the two-year mark.[8]

For the poor PWA there is a much more complicated array of available programs and services. PWAs whose income has been lost due to unemployment and who have no or few resources can apply for Supplemental Security Income (SSI). SSI requires both disability determination and low income. It pays a monthly cash assistance stipend, usually somewhat on the low side.[9] SSI carries with it automatic eligibility for Medicaid—the hospitalization and medical insurance for the needy. Those PWAs who have higher incomes or resource levels than allowed for SSI, but whose incurred medical expenses are high relative to their income, may still be able to receive Medicaid benefits. Coverage, especially for home care, is extended on a "spend down" basis (i.e., the PWA must apply a certain amount of his monthly income to medical or home care bills), Medicaid will pay the remainder.

In New York City, the Human Resources Administration (HRA) has attempted to expedite the processing of Medicaid applications for eligible PWAs in its Medical Assistance Program (MAP) Division. Additionally, the New York HRA has created AIDS Case Management Units to ensure comprehensive service provision to PWAs who are Medicaid-covered. Each PWA has a caseworker in a Case Management Unit who coordinates Medicaid-funded home care services, reviews his entitlement to other assistance and support services (for example, SSI, SSD, or food stamps), and negotiates any housing problems or disputes.[10]

These government assistance programs represent an admirable effort to address the social, medical, and economic needs of the financially poor PWA. However, the programs are often understaffed and overbureaucratized. Applicants for home care can wait weeks or months for a caseworker to be assigned to them. The paper work involved is intricate, time consuming, and entails coordination of input from PWA, doctor, caseworker, home care agencies, and others before care can be implemented. There is plenty of room for a snag to develop, and more often than not one or more miscommunications or misdeliveries of papers result in delay in the process. The PWA can await needed home care in the hospital and many who wait do so for months for no reason other than bureaucracy. Furthermore, for most professional individuals who are PWAs, the government's means-tested assistance programs with limited income requirements have minimal significance. Most are, for the duration of their illness, ineligible due to their higher income or resource levels.[11] While the professional may be eligible for SSD, this often takes so long to process that it is rendered meaningless, as the following case illustrates:

Bob received his first disability payment two weeks before he died. In the five months between application and receipt of benefits, his condition had deteriorated so that he could barely leave his bed. In that period he had never ceased worrying about how to pay his rent and bills. Now that he could with some ease allow himself some extras, there was little in the material realm that could provide much comfort. He dourly noted to the social worker that the public would not have to worry that he'd be spending "their money" injudiciously.

Bob's case is only one of a number of cases where SSD benefits were observed to arrive when the PWA was at or near death. While other disabilities may be able to withstand the months-long wait for benefits, AIDS requires quicker response if SSD is to be truly helpful.

## Public Health Department Programs

The majority of public health department funding has gone to AIDS research and prevention rather than to programs for treatment and care (Arno 1986a:21). There is, however, one major federally funded program of note for PWAs which is administered through each state's department of public health. This is the AIDS Drug Assistance Program (ADAP). ADAP derives from a federal emergency fund to assist PWAs in paying for the drug Retrovir. More commonly known as AZT (azidothymidine), Retrovir is the only Federal Drug Administration approved drug which has been shown to inhibit the replication of HIV. Retrovir is manufactured by Burroughs Wellcome and sells for about $8,000 per year. Its high cost, its rather toxic side effects, and the fact that Burroughs Wellcome holds a monopoly on its production have made it a highly controversial drug (Thomas and Fox 1987). ADAP provides free Retrovir on a means-tested basis to PWAs who cannot afford the drug, or whose insurance will not cover its purchase. Income levels for eligibility are comparatively high.[12] The program, however, has only minimal utility for most PWAs. Medicaid recipients are covered for Retrovir, as are most professionals who have adequate major medical policies or composite coverage including nominal cost drug programs.

### Voluntary Nonprofit Organizations

In the voluntary nonprofit sphere, programs range from special AIDS service components in established organizations such as the American Red Cross and Cancer Care to newly emergent mutual assistance groups of which the Gay Men's Health Crisis (GMHC) is the best known. The Red Cross will train a PWA's friends and family members in home care and provide transportation services to medical appointments. Cancer Care attends to the psychosocial needs of PWAs with lymphoma or Kaposi's sarcoma diagnoses with counseling and support groups. If the PWA can demonstrate financial need, Cancer Care will also cost-share transportation to medical appointments and home care services. Many mental health clinics and some family service organizations have begun to offer special service to PWAs. These are often provided under federal or corporate grants. While some programs reflect genuine efforts to serve PWAs, others appear to be more superficial. Personnel are given quick training in AIDS psychosocial dynamics and are sold as experts. In the voluntary, nonprofit arena (and, as will be discussed later, in the private sector sphere as well) AIDS is "in." There is a scramble to attain grant monies by agencies and organizations whose continued existence has always depended on their ability to tap whatever is in vogue at the federal-corporate funding level.[13]

Established agencies were not, however, the earliest voluntary organizations to service PWAs. As with the other major cities affected by the AIDS epidemic, New York City has seen the emergence of a number of community-based mutual assistance organizations. These are nonprofit in form and rely primarily on volunteer labor.[14] Historically, self-help and mutual assistance groups have developed, initially in any event, in response to the government's failure to adequately provide for the needs of a particular group. Specifically, these movements tend to arise among those for whom access to care and services is restricted due to racism, sexism, or class discrimination (Katz and Bender 1976:11; Gartner and Riessman 1979:6–7). It is not surprising then that the mutual assistance form of service provision has become central in attempts to cope with the social needs of PWAs.[15]

In New York City, the Gay Men's Health Crisis (GMHC) is the best-known of these community-based groups. GMHC was formed by a group of professional gay men in the early 1980s to address the social and health needs of the PWA. The rationale for formation of the group was not only that the government did not provide for the needs of gay men, but "because PWAs are frequently estranged from their families, the support systems that usually ameliorate the psychological reactions to dying may not be available" (Nichols and Ostrow 1984:78).

GMHC will provide services for all people with AIDS.[16] Services include crisis intervention counseling, a "buddy" program which assigns volunteers to help with daily living tasks, recreational programs, support and therapy groups, and legal, financial, and health care advocacy. Dunne (1987:677) reports that since incorporation [GMHC has] provided financial, legal, emotional and home care services to nearly 4,000 people with AIDS, or 15 percent of all AIDS cases in the United States, developed educational programs for the general public, for health care and social welfare professionals, and for homosexual and bisexual men that are models of their kind . . . and done this, at least initially with very little government support. . . . This is . . . an indictment of the social welfare and health care institutions that failed to respond to the AIDS epidemic.

Other voluntary nonprofit programs that have been formed within the gay community include the Lambda Legal and Educational Defense Fund and the PWA Coalition. The latter provides a number of social services, including meal programs, social groups, support groups, and "healing circles." The PWA Coalition publishes a monthly newsletter which updates readers on progress in both traditional and nontraditional treatment of AIDS, and contains a list of available services in New York and surrounding areas. These groups, along with other alternative health education and care groups such as HEAL and Northern Lights, attempt to connect PWAs with resources and support which the government has failed to supply.

GMHC, the PWA Coalition, and other such groups are indeed important resources for gay and bisexual PWAs. There does, however, appear to be class-related variation in the utilization of such organizations. GMHC services were often sought reluctantly or as a last resort by a number of the professionals with AIDS interviewed by the author. Other health care workers interviewed also reported they observed a trend away from use of community-based services among the clients that they had worked with. While the professionals with AIDS certainly acknowledged the value of such services for others, and on occasion would themselves serve as volunteers in these organizations, they often felt that they themselves had no need for the mutual assistance group services. This was in many cases true—the professional with AIDS relies primarily upon informal supports and on privately funded care. This is possible because, as will be discussed below, professionals have, for the most part, viable informal support networks functioning in conjunction with quite adequate health insurance provided through corporate or union group policy plans.

## INFORMAL SERVICES: THE SUPPORT OF FAMILY AND FRIENDS

As we have seen, formal services are less central to the illness experience of the professional with AIDS than for those who are less affluent. In lieu of formal supports, the professional appears to rely strongly on the combined efforts of family and friends.

For gay PWAs as a group, the viability and availability of familial support is often complicated by the fact that many are estranged from their families, or their families are geographically distant. Many PWAs initially moved to New

York to live in a less stigmatizing environment. Many have never directly discussed their personal lives with their families. In some cases, the families of those who have "come out" have broken off communication with the PWA. In fact, as mentioned earlier, one central reason for the formation of GMHC was the need for supports to replace those which might have in other cases been provided for the chronically ill patient by his family (Nichols and Ostrow 1984:78). It is indeed true that for many members of the gay community, networks of friends from career and social worlds have become surrogate family. One might expect, therefore, that the biological family would lose significance to the socially constructed family. While this may be the case for some, for most professionals with AIDS a less simple arrangement emerges—one involving support provision from both family and friends, but often with significant variation in the involvement of one group over the other relative to the stage of the disease.

The supportive role of the professional's friend network is most apparent in the early and middle stages of illness. Friends may be fewer due to death from AIDS, or constrained in the amount of time and energy they can spare due to work commitments. However, they often provide for most of the professional's support needs in the early months or years when the PWA is still able to retain some level of independence. Friends will pool their free time to help with daily household chores, setting up schedules among themselves for alternating shopping, cleaning, laundry, and so forth when the PWA is ill.[17] Friends will also provide temporary homes for PWAs who cannot, for example, return to their multifloor walkup apartments or remain alone while recuperating from an acute phase of the illness. Friends both help financially and advise in decision making around health care.

The role of friends in providing access to larger networks of information and assistance is particularly noteworthy. For the professional, problems with insurance, medical questions, legal issues, and transportation needs are often dealt with via manipulation of the various circles of people who intertwine in the professional network. In fact, it is through such networking as that described below that we can see how reliance on community-based services is replaced by professional class-specific behavior.

John, an educator, needed some legal advice about his medical insurance coverage. Rather than contact GMHC's legal department, he asked his friend Sally, a psychologist, if she knew someone in the legal field who might be able to help him. He had himself once referred Sally a private therapy client, so Sally "owed" him. Sally's friend Martha was married to a lawyer and Sally asked her if John might call her husband for some advice. Martha's husband was glad to help Sally who had in fact once referred him a private legal client.

In this case, John asked Sally for help within the context of an informal system of exchange with understood rules of reciprocity. Through such exchanges on an informal level, professionals are able to get what they need without enduring the stress of bureaucratic interactions and while maintaining some sense of personal independence.[18] So long as the resources remain available on an informal level, the professional with AIDS will prefer to use this route, as one PWA aptly described, to "call in my chits to get what I need."

The social and emotional costs of reliance on friends are however often not considered. The PWA's friends can provide only so much assistance before they begin to feel burdened and overwhelmed. Caring and support can become tinged with resentment and attendant feelings of guilt. Likewise, the PWA can only "receive" so much before he begins to feel too dependent. An ill PWA has limited ability to reciprocate. His active participation in a system of exchange can revert to a sense of helplessness, inadequacy, or depression. Reliance on friends and, as will be seen, on family over formal more impersonal sources of aid and assistance can take its toll.

While friends continue to offer support to the professional with AIDS throughout the course of the illness, there is often need for more full-time assistance as he becomes less able to function independently. Thus as the professional becomes more ill, we generally see greater family involvement. Although some of these men do indeed have estranged relationships with their families, it is almost universally observed that they do ultimately discuss their illness with their families who then contribute in some form and for some amount of time.

The reactions of the families to the situation vary. They may be angry, upset, or frightened of contagion risk.[19] While they may have some irrational fears about these issues, the families of professionals tend, however, to be well-educated about AIDS, the mode of transmission, and the lack of contagion risk associated with care and casual contact.[20] Unlike poorer families such as those discussed by Honey (1988), Hopkins (1987), and Mays and Cochran (1987), families of these professionals are more able to provide money, time, and housing space for their ill sons or brothers. Most families observed in the author's work with PWAs did respond to their relative's illness. Contributions ranged from money to housing to hands-on personal care support. Involvement was most often at the request and with the approval of the PWA. In fact, many of these PWAs preferred to return to their family homes to die. Families most often supported this desire.[21] The wish to return to the family home may not itself be class-specific. However, the possibility of such a move is strongly class related. It depends not only on the family's fact-based understanding of the illness, but on the objective conditions of a family's socioeconomic status. As Honey (1988:387) points out, "Poor, ethnic minority families frequently live in overcrowded housing conditions and may not have space for the nonambulatory, debilitated PWA who needs constant care."

Returning home or otherwise relying on the family can entail certain costs, however. Family involvement is often characterized by the setting of informal, generally unspoken conditions. While the family might not express the conditions directly to their son or brother, he is often aware of the subtleties of

the contract. Families will be there so long as their own "name" is not compromised, and so long as the privacy of personal family affairs is respected by
the PWA and his friends. For example, families of PWAs and the professionals
themselves often agree to explain the illness to other family and friends as
"cancer" or "pneumonia." Likewise, the PWA may "decide" to return home
with only certain kinds of treatments, especially those not requiring extensive
visiting nurse care or public health department scrutiny. Such treatments might
include intravenous antibiotics like amphotericin which requires continuous
nursing presence during the infusion due to toxic side effects, or drugs which
require blood tests to monitor anemia levels and other side effects. Families
often fear that outside agency involvement will lead to gossip and non-familial
access to information about the PWA's true medical status. Although agency
files are confidential, neighbors might see vans or health care personnel entering
the home and "begin to talk." While they themselves accept him, families
doubt—sometimes with reason—that others will be so broad-minded about
AIDS. Families can be especially concerned when there are younger children
who might be vulnerable to chiding from schoolmates.

This sensitivity to family fears about what others might think of their connection with a PWA was also in certain cases explanatory of the professional's
reluctance to utilize community-based organizations. For PWAs who wish to
have a closer connection to their family, who are indicating some ambivalence
about their son's gayness or bisexuality, involvement with GMHC, for example,
was often avoided. Such an association would align the PWA with the stigmatized population that his family wishes to avoid. Families can subtly set up
a dichotomous situation of either "that world will take care of you, or we will."
The ill PWA who wishes to maintain family support will rarely challenge this.

The price of family involvement can at times go beyond such compromises
into causing disruption in the support from friends. Although family and friends
may predominate at different times as primary support givers, the reality is that
for most professionals both groups together comprise the informal network of
support. Thus conflict between family and friends can be a major problem. The
following case exemplifies this.

John was in the final stages of his illness when his parents became involved. They had
not been closely involved in his adult life—in fact had not known that he was living a
gay life-style until his diagnosis a year before. It was a difficult revelation for them, and
it was hard for them at times to separate their anxieties about the life-style of their son
from the fears around his illness. They however pushed their many reactions into the
background as John's condition deteriorated and rallied to his hospital bedside in the
final weeks of his illness. In the early months following his diagnosis, John had appointed
his lover Jim his power of attorney should this be necessary and executor of his will.
This was difficult for John's father who felt the family should be responsible for John's
affairs. Furthermore, while John's parents knew that the feeling was irrational, they
couldn't help but blame Jim for John's illness or wonder why John and not Jim was lying
in the hospital bed dying. As John became sicker, tensions between John's father and

Jim grew to such an extent that John's father hired an attorney to contest John's appointment of Jim as executor and power of attorney. Legal battling involved doctor and hospital staff as well as family and friends. Both Jim and the family tried to keep John from knowing about the conflict, but he noticed his lover's absence and the tension in his family when he asked where Jim was.

Most situations are not so strained as that depicted above. While there may be an undercurrent of stress, both parties work to contain feelings that might upset their ill relative or friend. In many cases such as the following, family and friends manage to combine forces in the interest of the PWA's care needs.

Billy lived with his lover Will for the first few years of his illness. During the final hospitalization, Will and Billy's parents took turns staying with Billy. Billy's parents spoke highly of Will and appeared to get along with him. As Billy's condition stabilized, planning began for him to return home with Will. One day, as discharge approached, Billy announced that plans had changed. He was going to his parents' home. When I asked Will why his plans had changed, he responded with a shrug, "His parents said I'd had him with me for three years and that was enough . . . that it was their turn now to have him with them."

Rather than splintering the support network as the conflict between Jim and John's family had done, however, Billy's family invited Will to spend weekends and extra time with them. For Billy, this significantly eased the transition to his parents' home.

Conflicts and strains within the support network can be most disturbing for the PWA not only because of his emotional connection to both friends and family, but because his social well-being often depends on the successful articulation of both groups as support providers. Alienation of one group leaves him feeling more vulnerable to the potential loss of the other. Reliance on informal levels of support may result in lower economic costs but can demand varied social and emotional returns from all parties. Calculating the "cost of care" for the professional PWA obviously entails much more than tabulating medical and hospital bills.

## PRIVATE SECTOR SERVICES: HOME CARE AND THE CHRONICALLY-ACUTE PATIENT

Class variation in the experience of AIDS is most clearly manifest in access to and utilization of home care services, especially those provided by private profit-making agencies. Home care can involve skilled nursing care, the monitoring of intravenous drug infusions, social work services, occupational and physical therapy, home health aide care, housekeeping services, and meal delivery. The importance of home care in the spectrum of AIDS-related services derives from the way in which the specific character of the AIDS disease process has dovetailed with recent trends in health care delivery in this country.

AIDS is both a chronic and acute disease which may take a different course for each PWA. Some maintain fairly normal lives for months or even years before hospitalization. Others may go through periods of severe illness but rebound to levels of fairly independent self-care. Depending upon the opportunistic infections present, the illness may also progress slowly or rapidly and be more or less debilitating. Persons with AIDS enter hospitals with such acute conditions as pneumonia and meningitis but often leave needing care for chronic conditions such as colitis, progressive blindness, and HIV-related dementia.

Combining both chronic and acute states, AIDS enters a health care system which had developed around the acute care needs of the middle-aged male and is floundering in its attempts to serve its present primary users, the chronically-ill aging female population (see Sidel and Sidel 1977:44–46; Fox 1986). Since insurance would cover hospital care, these institutions, designed for acute care, were by the 1960s and 1970s becoming havens for the chronically ill, especially those with cancer for whom there were few affordable alternate care options. This situation, combined with developments in medical technology, led to extensive outlays by both private insurance companies and the Medicare/Medicaid insurance programs. In the ensuing attempts to restructure the health care system, home care became targeted as the answer to the sky-rocketing insurance costs. Changes were made in Medicare in 1982 in an attempt to remediate the gap in chronic care delivery. Limited home care coverage for the aged was added, accompanied by a cap on hospital stay spending. Private insurance companies soon followed suit in extending the amount of coverage for home care (Burke and Koren 1984). This spurred on efforts by health care providers to respond to the new market and has resulted in a continued growth in revenues for the home health care industry.

The feasibility of home care as an option for any chronic care patient depends on the presence of three interlocking factors. First, the home care tool kit must contain adequate medical technology for the patient's care needs. Second, there must be financial resources, adequate insurance coverage or both to pay for what can be quite costly services. Third, as Burke and Koren (1984:9) point out,

The most important and least obvious aspect of the home care service sector is the patient's personal support system. In most cases it is a patient's family and friends who provide essential services to homebound patients. The presence or absence of a primary caregiver in the home often determines whether home care is a viable option.

As will be discussed below, all these factors converge nicely in the case of the professional with AIDS.

Home medical care needs for the PWA can range from a need for brief nursing visits and home health aide services to high-tech care involving complexly timed intravenous drug infusions and intravenous nutritional supports. While in the early 1980s this kind of care was of limited availability for the home patient, in recent years high-tech equipment has become more accessible, especially in the more urban areas of the country. In fact, high-tech home care sales are increasing at enormous rates (Roe and Schneider 1985:52; Barhydt-Wezenaar 1986; Haddad 1987). There is very little medical care that might be required for the PWA which theoretically could not be provided at home, including both equipment and the personnel trained in its use. Such care, is, however, quite expensive. Costs for 24 hours of home nursing care can be $600 or more per day. Equipment and supplies for the simplest intravenous drug infusion common in the treatment of AIDS-related infections can cost $75 per day.

The Medicaid program will furnish certain types of home care in New York City. It does not reimburse private agency care, however, but only that directly provided by or subcontracted through the Visiting Nurse Service.[22] As reported increasingly by the news media, Medicaid recipients and those who are applying for Medicaid-funded home care often spend endless months in hospitals merely awaiting the implementation of publicly funded home care services (Lambert 1989). There is a significant scarcity of home care workers in New York City and finding those willing to work with PWAs is a continued problem (Iverem 1988). When combined with the bureaucratic snags that plague the Medicaid process, the attempt to get home care through Medicaid is, as the following case exemplifies, a frustrating endeavor for the Medicaid eligible PWA.

George had applied for Medicaid-funded home care in mid-August. It was early September before his application was completed and docked in at MAP. While he was quickly assigned a Medicaid number denoting funding eligibility, it was mid-October before he was assigned a caseworker. By mid-November the application for home care specifically had not been completed. The caseworker had visited George in the hospital, had visited his home to assess care needs there and had submitted a number of required forms in that period of time, but had not received any notification from the Home Care Division of MAP regarding approval for home care. As it was considered medically unsafe for him to go home without care, George had been waiting in the hospital. However, with family and friends agreeing to work out a schedule of care for a temporary period of time, he decided to go home, knowing that he might wait indefinitely for home care to be implemented through the Medicaid bureaucracy. Soon after George went home, it came to our attention that his home care application had been relayed to the wrong office and had remained dormant for two weeks. Finally, in early December, after a four-month long process, he was evaluated and eligible for home care. However, by late December there was still no care in place due to a lack of home health aides available for work with PWAs in his borough of New York City. By this time George, his family, and friends were at the edge of their emotional endurance. George was depressed and his medical condition was deteriorating.

The Medicaid Home Care Division can furthermore reject more complicated home care cases, such as one in which the PWA might require continuous nursing care. Medicaid programs are understaffed and nursing hours must be used economically. When a number of patients could be serviced with the hours used in the care of one, such a patient would best be left in an institutional setting. Indeed, it is mainly those for whom home care is not a viable option due to either lack of domicile, complexity of care needs, or minimal support system who swell the ranks of the "unplaceable"—those for whom terminal care facilities or nursing home beds have yet to be provided in New York City.[23]

Those who can remain outside the Medicaid system of services and who can purchase care from private agencies either because of insurance coverage or available resources can have many more options. For the less affluent, buying private home care would be unthinkable due to the excessive cost. However, the professional with AIDS tends to be covered by group health insurance obtained through employment, by and large a kind of health insurance that has comparatively thorough major medical components that will cover extensive home care services. Private sector profit-making programs are increasingly becoming a major provider of home care services to this population and some are doing it quite effectively as compared with other purveyors of assistance. In fact, a number of agencies have formed special AIDS divisions. Such care is often more expensive than that provided by regular home care agencies, but this is rationalized by the fact that staff are trained to have better knowledge of the complexities of AIDS care.

The private insurance company has been especially eager to develop and finance home care options for PWAs despite the cost. The average hospital care cost in New York City is nearly $1,000 per day. Home care costs can be one-quarter to one-half of that of care in a hospital. Needless to say, insurers are often more than willing to go to great lengths to support home care for PWAs (Oppenheimer and Padgug 1986).[24]

The insurance coverage of the professional with AIDS dovetails with aspects of the support environment of the professional population to yield a situation ripe for private sector involvement. First, as mentioned earlier, families tend to be supportive of the PWA but to also have certain conditions around their support. Of importance is the desire for privacy and governmental health or social service agency involvement in family affairs threatens the family's sense of privacy about the AIDS-related circumstances with which they are confronted. The preference for private sector care, even when insurance will *not* cover this, has been a characteristic of these families, some of whom can and will manage to pay for private sector care even if it means selling homes or taking out loans.[25]

Family structure supplements this desire for privacy in reinforcing the trend toward privately hired home care. It is notable that these families of a professional with AIDS characteristically consist of adult children and parents who are just at retirement age. Parents are thus old enough to not be working, but young enough to be able to take on some of the responsibility of care. Strictly speaking, they could be available for supervision of home care agency personnel and for running errands should the PWA wish to stay with his parents at home. As noted earlier, friends and lovers are often available for similar purposes for the PWA who does not return to live with his family. Effective home care entails the need for social supports, and this both family and friends can often provide.

For the professional with AIDS then, the basic components for a viable home care plan can exist fairly easily in most cases. While this allows for more care options, it has in the past few years also rendered them subject to home care agency marketeering. More and more, profit-making home care agencies are targeting service to the professional with AIDS as a money-making endeavor. Personnel of some of the more popular private home care agencies working with New York PWAs have become adept at public relations, at sensitivity to the desire for confidentiality and, most importantly, at advocating with insurance companies for extended home care benefits for the PWA. Should someone skilled in the costs and processes of third-party payment attempt this, most insurance companies can be convinced that it will be cheaper to enlarge on a policy's provisions than to have an insuree hospitalized. For the PWA who needs home care and wants to be out of the hospital as soon as his medical condition allows, the private agency can arrange quality home care with a minimum, if any, delay. Unlike George's experience, the professional with good insurance can request home service one day and have it the next.

This is a strong selling point to a PWA who wishes to be at home, or to families and friends who may be burdened themselves to provide adequate care for the PWA. Obviously, the private agency has more than the client's interests in view in providing such efficient services. But in a city where requests for services for PWAs are often answered with, "We don't know if we can find someone to work with an AIDS patient," PWAs and their networks are not inclined to question motivations.

While options in care and treatment such as those described above are certainly to be welcomed, they often bring with them even more intricate choices— ones that reveal the entanglement of AIDS care and treatment in what Waitzkin and Waterman (1974) term the health care industry's "exploitation of illness." Marketeering by home care agencies is as blatant a form of exploitation as the failure to provide adequate home care for the Medicaid recipient. That treatment and care resulting in the prolongation of life are more available to the insured than to the noninsured is a fact. But providing equal access to all, while important, has resulted less in a diminution of suffering than in the expansion of markets for pharmaceutical companies and a fueling of competition within the home health care industry. In a capitalist society, access does not rule out exploitation. A more subtle form of exploitation lies in the questionable prolongation and enlargement of suffering on the emotional as well as physical levels that accompanies the particular pattern of service distribution. And while the professional with AIDS may not have to worry about home care availability, he does have to contend more directly with whether his family really wants to house him, and whether going with his family will result in a curtailment of his friends' support. While the professional may not have to worry about access to the newest intravenous therapeutic drug, he does have to take on questions about whether, because a company has an antibiotic to test, he wants to endure more toxic side effects or to have his life prolonged in light of his progressing blindness. Where economic access is less the question, the deeper dimensions of the health care system's exploitation of illness are more apparent.

## CONCLUSION

For gay and bisexual PWAs in New York City, class has become a major organizer of the illness experience. Reflecting a general theme of provision of assistance only to those who are of desperately low income, governmental programs are geared primarily to the needy AIDS population. Voluntary nonprofit and community-based services and programs are available to all, but used less by the professional with AIDS who relies mainly on informal networks of family and friends for care and support. For the professional, family support engenders a heightened emphasis on privacy which reinforces the trend away from utilization of community-based care and toward involvement with private home care agency services. This trend is underwritten by the professional's access to extensive major medical insurance coverage which makes him a sought-after market for the burgeoning home health care industry.

Reliance on informal supports and private care dramatically distinguishes the professional's experience of AIDS from that of the less affluent. For the latter, the objective course of the illness is reportedly locked in struggles around housing, public assistance bureaucracies, and actual access to medical care support services. The professional with AIDS is confronted with a different set of problems. Once presented with options by virtue of resources or insurance coverage, the emotional and social costs of continuing to live with AIDS become more apparent.

Class variation in the experience of AIDS such as that described here can be missed in focusing upon the "risk group." If we wish to understand the reality of AIDS so as to provide a more humane context for treatment and care for all, we may benefit from attending to the dynamics of the illness in relation to more culturally germane groups such as class, family, or ethnic group.

## NOTES

An earlier version of this chapter was presented at the Annual Meeting of the Northeastern Anthropological Association in Albany, N.Y., March 1988. I wish to thank the staff of New York University Medical Center's Department of Social Work for their information and support. I am also grateful to Shellee Colen and Richard Blot for their editorial help. This chapter is dedicated to the memory of Robert Golden.

1. "In-kind" services are concrete, nonmonetary forms of aid (e.g., free housing, free food, or specific services) granted to individuals in need.

2. The definition of social services as comprising only *formal*-level services is an essentially sociological definition which fails to address the ideological and behavioral

complexity of modern life. As Eric Wolf (1966:2) states below, the totality of the cultural scenario of modern life cannot be reduced to formal structures:

[T]he formal framework of economic and political power exists alongside intermingled with various other kinds of informal structures which are interstitial, supplementary, parallel to it. . . . Sometimes such informal groupings cling to the formal structure like barnacles to a rusty ship. At other times, informal social relations are responsible for the metabolic processes required to keep the formal institution operative. . . . In still other cases, we discover that the formal table of organization is elegant indeed, but fails to work, unless informal mechanisms are found for its direct contravention.

3. Recently a number of authors have begun to address the variation within the AIDS experience that is engendered by minority group membership. See, for example Honey 1988; Friedman et al. 1987; Hopkins 1987; and Mays and Cochran 1987. While these studies are a move toward a more refined understanding of the AIDS problem in the United States, as Moynihan et al. (1988:381) and Finney (1987:19) point out, "minority group" is an ideologically laden social class and regional distinction which renders those in that group as questionable as a risk group in focusing on commonality of experience. What these authors appear to be in fact discussing is the effects of poverty on the AIDS experience. Torres, Lefkowitz et al. (1987) who focus on homelessness as the significant factor affecting both medical and social welfare of PWAs, and Finney (1987), stand out in their direct attention to class issues.

4. See, for example, Drucker (1986) for a discussion of "drug culture" among intravenous drug users.

5. This group mirrors what statistics reveal to be the most characteristic group of PWAs in New York City at present, that is, male homosexuals and bisexuals between the ages of 30 and 50 comprise over 6,000 of the over 14,000 PWAs in New York (New York City Department of Health 1988:7).

6. Information on nonprofessional PWAs is taken from the literature cited in note 3 above, direct clinical social work with PWAs, and material from interviews with health care workers. The latter two sources were less extensively relied on, however, than information on the professionals who are the major focus of this study.

7. A diagnosis of AIDS automatically entitles eligibility for disability status for SSD. Those with AIDS-related conditions (ARC), however, must still establish disability status through the normal, often lengthy, channels. See U.S. Department of Health (1987:6–25) for review of disability benefits for PWAs.

8. See Andrulis et al. (1987a:1345; 1987b) for discussion of hospitalization payment sources for PWAs in private vs. public hospitals. Medicaid coverage is accepted by fewer doctors due to its low reimbursement rates. Therefore fewer PWAs are admitted to private hospitals which are preferred because of their reputations for higher quality medical care. Medicare coverage is, however, standardly accepted by most doctors. Provision of Medicare to PWAs would make private hospital admissions more possible and would allow for more treatment options.

9. SSI was instituted to provide a minimum income level for the aged, blind, and disabled. The payment is subject to what is termed a "less eligibility" requirement, meaning that the amount the recipient is paid must be slightly below what a working citizen would earn in a month's period of time. The underpinning ideology is one of encouraging work over welfare.

10. In New York City, Medicaid eligibility brings with it qualification for the few

publicly funded AIDS housing programs, that is, Bailey House and Scattered Site Housing.

11. For some PWAs, private insurance is used for coverage in the earlier period of the illness until resources are exhausted or care needs extend beyond that provided by private insurance at which time they become Medicaid eligible. These PWAs who shift from private insurance to Medicaid are difficult to locate in statistics on payment sources for AIDS care (see Luehrs et al. 1986:21). The complexity of source of payment for AIDS care is enhanced by the fact that through the Consolidated Omnibus Budget Reconciliation Act of 1985 (COBRA), many PWAs have the opportunity to continue for 18 months with their private group policy coverage after leaving their employment. Families will often pay for this coverage to retain care options for the PWA. See Borzi (1987) and Fulginiti (1987) for a discussion of COBRA insurance coverage provisions.

12. In New York State, eligibility for ADAP in 1988 carried income limits of $22,000 for a single-person household and $29,600 for a two-person household. For discussion and critique of public funding for AIDS research and services, see Arno (1986a; 1986b) and Krieger (1988).

13. Wells (1987) reviews trends in corporate foundation funding for AIDS research and care.

14. See Arno (1988; 1986b) for his important economic analysis of the utilization of volunteer labor in community-based services for PWAs in both New York City and San Francisco.

15. Arno (1986a:24) providess a succinct analysis of government support for community-based organizations staffed by volunteer labor: "What is taking place is a shifting of costs from federal to state and local governments and on to individuals."

16. Arno (1988:9) notes differential utilization of GMHC services. However,

During the first six months of 1987, GMHC added to its caseload an average of 47 percent, 13 percent and 17 percent of the city's newly diagnosed AIDS cases among whites, blacks and Hispanics, respectively. These figures indicate that whites are much more likely to be served by GMHC than blacks or Hispanics, and furthermore, that the increasing spread of AIDS among these groups has not been matched by increased service demands at GMHC.

17. One major problem often emerges in the professional's network around the fact that friends in social circles often do not know friends in career circles. A commonly observed solution to this dilemma was the "network organizer"—a friend who will survey the PWA's phone book with him and take responsibility for contacting people and setting up the assistance schedule.

18. Wills (1985) offers an interesting discussion isolating the functions of social support. Despite the fact that friends might not be directly available for the professional with AIDS at times, their ability to provide contact with sources of assistance, to access information or to "break through" bureaucracies because of their professional status makes them quite valuable.

19. See Stulberg and Buckingham (1988) for a description of issues commonly faced by families of PWAs.

20. The value placed on education is noted by Ehrenreich and Ehrenreich (1979) in their definition of the professional-managerial class. Furthermore, professional families may be both better educated about and more inclined to accept a scientific stand favoring lack of contagion risk than the less affluent (see Honey 1988:367 and Hopkins 1987:679).

21. See Droste (1987) for a consideration of the economic and social problems engendered in local public health care by the move toward "dying at home."

22. The Visiting Nurse Service of New York (VNS) is certified to receive Medicaid and Blue Cross reimbursement. Most private agencies are licensed but not specifically certified by the state in this manner.

23. Lambert (1989:B2) reports:

[New York State's] first nursing home ward for AIDS was originally scheduled to open in Manhattan in October [1988]. But the opening has been delayed until early this year [1989]. Two other AIDS nursing homes and a third health-related facility are also proposed this year. If they materialize, they would raise the total capacity to 364 beds.

Existing nursing homes have been reluctant to take PWAs because they claim they are not adequately reimbursed for the extensive care necessary. There is a limited number of beds available for PWAs at Goldwater Memorial Hospital on Roosevelt Island. This is a city facility similar to a nursing home which provides chronic care services.

24. Oppenheimer and Padgug (1986:20) point out,

AIDS and ARC strike primarily males between the ages of twenty and fifty, precisely the classes that are most often found in employee health insurance groups—the most common form of private health insurance—and that, until now, have had the lowest rates of health utilization . . . AIDS seems to strike directly at the heart of the principles of "sound underwriting" that underlie private health insurance. Given a sufficiently high incidence, the disease might, many believe, make private reimbursement for AIDS treatment impossible.

25. Using private medical/health care facilities to avoid public exposure of mental illness, pregnancy, and other stigmatized conditions is a well-documented phenomenon associated with higher socioeconomic groups. See, for example, Ryan (1976:99–101).

# REFERENCES

Andrulis, Dennis P., et al. 1987a. The Provision and Financing of Medical Care of AIDS Patients in U.S. Public and Private Teaching Hospitals. *Journal of the American Medical Association* 258:1343–46.

———. 1987b. State Medicaid Policies and Hospital Care for AIDS Patients. *Health Affairs* 6:10–118.

Arno, Peter S. 1988. The Future of Voluntarism and the AIDS Epidemic. Unpublished paper delivered at Cornell University Medical Conference: The AIDS Patient—An Action Agenda for New York City, February 25, 1988.

———. 1986a. AIDS: A Balancing Act of Resources. *Business and Health* 4:20–24.

———. 1986b. The Nonprofit Sector's Response to the AIDS Epidemic: Community Based Services in San Francisco. *American Journal of Public Health* 76:1325–30.

Barhydt-Wezenaar, Nancy. 1986. Home Care and Hospice. In *Health Care Delivery in the United States*, Steven Jonas, ed., pp. 237–62. New York: Springer.

Borzi, Phyllis C. 1987. What does COBRA Portend for the Future? *Business and Health* 5:4–6.

Burke, Gregory C., and Mary Jane Koren. 1984. Home Care: An Industry on the Horizon. *Business and Health* 2:8–13.

Droste, Therese. 1987. Going Home to Die: Developing Home Health Care Services for AIDS Patients. *Hospitals* (August):54–58.

Drucker, Ernest. 1986. AIDS and Addiction in New York City. *American Journal of Drug and Alcohol Abuse* 12:165–81.

Dunne, Richard D. 1987. AIDS in New York City: Policy and Planning. *Bulletin of the New York Academy of Medicine* 63:673–78.

Ehrenreich, Barbara, and John Ehrenreich. 1979. The Professional-Managerial Class and Rejoinder. In *Between Labor and Capital*, Pat Walker, ed., pp. 5–48 and 313–34. Boston: South End Press.

Finney, Angus. 1987. What Are Poor Folk to Do? *New Statesman* 113, 2921:19–20.

Fox, Daniel M. 1986. AIDS and the American Health Polity: The History and Prospects of a Crisis of Authority. *The Milbank Quarterly* 64:7–33.

Friedman, Samuel R., et al. 1987. The AIDS Epidemic Among Blacks and Hispanics. *The Milbank Quarterly* 65:455–99.

Fulginiti, Mari P. 1987. An Employer's Assessment of Continuation Coverage. *Business and Health* 5:8–11.

Gartner, Alan, and Frank Riessman. 1979. *Selfhelp in the Human Services*. San Francisco: Jossey Bass.

Haddad, Amy Marie. 1987. *High Tech Home Care: A Practical Guide*. Rockville, Maryland: Aspen Publishers.

Honey, Ellen. 1988. AIDS and the Inner City: Critical Issues. *Social Casework* 69:365–70.

Hopkins, Donald R. 1987. AIDS in Minority Populations in the United States. *Public Health Reports* 102:677–81.

Iverem, Esther. 1988. New York's Home Health Care System Facing a Labor Crisis. *New York Times*, January 28, p. B1.

Katz, Alfred, and Eugene I. Bender, eds. 1976. *The Strength in Us: Self Help Groups in the Modern World*. New York: New Viewpoints.

Krieger, Nancy. 1988. AIDS Funding: Competing Needs and the Politics of Priorities. *International Journal of Health Services* 18:521–41.

Lambert, Bruce. 1989. In Spite of Crisis, New York Lacks Basic Services for AIDS Patients. *New York Times*, January 3, pp. A1, B2.

Luehrs, John, Evagreen Orlebeke, and Mark Merles. 1986. AIDS and Medicaid. *Public Welfare* 44, 3:20–28.

Mays, Vickie M., and Susan D. Cochran. 1987. Acquired Immunodeficiency Syndrome and Black Americans: Special Psychosocial Issues. *Public Health Reports* 102:224–31.

Moynihan, Rosemary, Grace Christ, and Les Gallo Silver. 1988. AIDS and Terminal Illness. *Social Casework* 69:380–87.

New York City Department of Health, AIDS Surveillance Unit. 1988. *AIDS Surveillance Update*, September 28.

Nichols, Stuart E., and David Ostrow, eds. 1984. *Psychiatric Implications of Acquired Immune Deficiency Syndrome*. Washington, D.C.: American Psychiatric Press.

Oppenheimer, Gerald M., and Robert A. Padgug. 1986. AIDS: The Risks to Insurers, the Threat to Equity. *Hastings Center Report* 16:18–22.

Roe, Wayne I., and Gary S. Schneider. 1985. High-Tech Moves into Home Market with Cardiac, Nutritional Therapies. *Business and Health* 2:52–53.

Ryan, William. 1976. *Blaming the Victim*. New York: Random House/Vintage.

Sidel, Victor, and Ruth Sidel. 1977. *A Healthy State: An International Perspective on the Crisis in United States Medical Care*. New York: Pantheon.

Stack, Carol. 1974. *All Our Kin: Strategies for Survival in a Black Community*. New York: Harper and Row.

Stulberg, Ian, and Stephen L. Buckingham. 1988. Parallel Issues for AIDS Patients, Families, and Others. *Social Casework* 69:355–59.

Thomas, Emily, and Daniel M. Fox. 1987. The Cost of AZT. *AIDS and Public Policy Journal* 2:17–21.

Torres, Ramon A., Pearl Lefkowitz et al. 1987. Homelessness Among Hospitalized Patients with the Acquired Immunodeficiency Syndrome in New York City. *Journal of the American Medical Association* 258:779–80.

U.S. Departmental of Health and Human Services/Public Health Department. 1987. AIDS: A Public Health Challenge; State Issues, Policies and Programs. Volume 2. *Managing and Financing the Problem*.

Waitzkin, Howard, and Barbara Waterman. 1974. *The Exploitation of Illness in Capitalist Society*. Indianapolis, Indiana: Bobbs-Merrill.

Weissman, Harold H. 1983. The Social Welfare System. In *The Human Services Delivery System*, S. Richard Sauber, ed., pp. 184–222. New York: Columbia University Press.

Wells, James A. 1987. Foundation Funding for AIDS Programs. *Health Affairs* 6:113–23.

Wills, Thomas Ashby. 1985. Supportive Functions of Interpersonal Relationships. In *Social Support and Health*, Sheldon Cohen and S. Leonard Syme, eds., pp. 61–82. Orlando: Academic Press.

Wolf, Eric. 1966. *Kinship, Friendship, and Patron-Client Relations in Complex Societies*, Michael Banton, ed., pp. 1–22. New York: Praeger.

# Chapter Thirteen

## Postscript: Anthropology and AIDS

### Douglas A. Feldman

Anthropologists have been involved in AIDS-related research and activities since the early 1980s. Today, there is the AIDS and Anthropology Research Group, with about 120 members, which produces a quarterly newsletter, holds national and regional meetings, and serves as a channel for the sharing of information by anthropologists working on AIDS. The American Anthropological Association has also appointed 23 anthropologists to form the AAA Task Force on AIDS. The Task Force is lobbying the United States Congress for AIDS-related funding, is preparing to review international AIDS policy from an anthropological perspective, is developing a teaching manual on AIDS and anthropology, and is preparing a special publication on the anthropology of AIDS. The International Commission on the Anthropology of AIDS was formed in 1988, and is based in Switzerland.

Anthropologists, as we have seen by the chapters in this volume, have engaged in a wide variety of AIDS-related activities and research projects. Anthropologists have conducted research analyzing sociocultural processes and change, have indeed become AIDS health educators, have become social workers for persons with AIDS, have conducted AIDS-related epidemiologic research, have used a remote sensing laboratory to map HIV patterns with cultural behavior, and have served as administrators for AIDS programs and community-based organizations. Indeed, the wide range of roles which anthropologists have assumed in our struggle against AIDS leads one inevitably to the question: Is there a *unique* role for anthropologists in AIDS-related research and activities?

Anthropologists, it is maintained here, can offer both a unique methodological approach to research and a unique conceptual framework for understanding the pandemic on a global level. Ethnography is the basic research method of cultural anthropologists (see Trotter 1988). It includes direct observation, participant observation, open-ended interviewing, and maintaining detailed field notes. Ethnographers directly observe what people in a culture or subculture do, in order to distinguish between what people actually do and what they think they do or what they say they do. Direct observation may include the physical setting, social interactions, or individual behavior.

Participant observation is often an important component of an ethnography, and involves interacting with members of the culture or subculture being studied. The ethnographer participates, at least to a limited degree, in the routine activities and special events of the people under study.

Open-ended interviewing includes casual conversations, probing questioning, the collection of life histories, the utilization of key informants, and conducting life cycle interviews. It is important to ascertain the attitudes, values, norms, and expectations of people in a culture or subculture. Open-ended interviewing permits the ethnographer to determine what is going on in the mind of the person being interviewed; it is not highly structured and allows for exploration into areas where there is little prior information. The increasing use of focus groups represents one form of open-ended interviewing that may be very useful as a supplement to basic ethnography.

Ethnographic research methods require maintaining highly detailed field notes. Ethnography demands very careful recording—on paper, on tape, and into computers. It is qualitative, descriptive research, and is subject to numerous ethical and security considerations. Ethnography may be used in conjunction with other research techniques, such as closed-ended interviewing, question-naires, utilizing census data, and using transcripts for linguistic analysis.

Ethnography is indispensable in discerning the parameters of social behavior, in understanding the sociocultural context, and in generating hypotheses. As we have seen, anthropologists have conducted, and are conducting, a number of important AIDS-related ethnographic studies. In addition to the material presented in this volume, other contributions include the following: Dr. Joseph Carrier, a consultant for the Orange County, California Department of Health, has been conducting open-ended interviewing and ethnographic field work among Mexican-American men who engage in homosexual behavior. He has found that many such men are not gay-identified even if they only have sex with other men and never with women. One defines himself as gay or homosexual only if he engages in receptive anal intercourse. Risk-reduction workshops targeted to homosexual Mexican-American men need to take this into account (Carrier and Magana 1989).

Monette Sachs, an anthropology doctoral candidate at Yale University, is conducting ethnographic fieldwork among persons with AIDS in New York City. She has found that the health care and social services systems are not working well in that city for most PWAs. They spend long hours waiting for services in the clinics at municipal hospitals. Many are homeless, suffer from poor nutrition, and their social networks are inadequate to meet their many needs. Dr. Ralph Bolton, of Pomona College in California, has used ethnographic methods in Belgium to determine that many gay men who are highly aware of safer sex practices do *not* engage in these risk-reduction techniques.

Dr. Janet McGrath, Dr. Debra Schumann, both of Case Western Reserve University in Cleveland, and Dr. Maxine Ankrah, of Makerere University in Uganda, have begun a family impact study of Ugandan families with AIDS using ethnographic methods to assess their needs and to understand the socio-cultural processes which occur within such households. Professor Sandra Wallman, a consultant for the British Medical Council, has begun an ethnological study on Ugandan cultures, sexual behavior, and AIDS.

Dr. Richard Parker and Carlos Coimbra, Jr., have been independently conducting fieldwork in Brazil among gay men to better understand the measures needed to develop a successful risk-reduction program. In addition to the work described in this volume by Dr. Sophie Day in London, England, Dr. Michele Schedlin in Bridgeport, Connecticut, and Terri Leonard in Camden, New Jersey, have conducted fieldwork among female prostitutes in those cities.

Many other anthropologists have also been involved in qualitative AIDS research. Recently, the National Institute of Drug Abuse (NIDA) near Washington, D.C., and Narcotics and Drug Research, Inc. (NDRI) in New York City have employed anthropologists or funded projects with anthropologists to better understand the sociocultural dynamics of intravenous drug use behavior and to evaluate approaches to risk reduction and to explore the meaning of risk-taking behavior. In addition to Dr. Dooley Worth, Doug Goldsmith, Dr. Theresa Mason, and Dr. Stephanie Kane are some of the anthropologists working in this area.

However, NIDA and NDRI are the rare exceptions. Few international and United States federal agencies have so far employed anthropologists to conduct AIDS-related ethnographic studies. Such research is urgently needed, especially if directed toward analyses of sexual behavior, belief systems, social networks and interaction, and evaluative assessment of risk-reduction programs. This kind of research is most needed among gay and bisexual men and among families with HIV infection in both developed and developing nations.

International and United States federal agencies bear the responsibility to bring anthropologists into their AIDS-related research projects and evaluations and to add an ethnographic component where necessary. Anthropologists, for our part, have a responsibility to see to it that the short-term ethnography is completed in a timely manner, or if it is a long-term ethnography, that periodic reports are written and published well before the conclusion of the study. Moreover, the research focus preferably should be problem-oriented and not designed to resolve strictly theoretical issues in social science research. We are in the midst of a grave global pandemic, and our research must be both useful and timely.

In addition to the contribution of ethnographic fieldwork, anthropologists can offer a unique conceptual framework for understanding AIDS from a very broad perspective. To the cultural anthropologist, all cultures, all ways of human life, have intrinsic value and worth, regardless of the population size of the culture or its apparent uniqueness. The Ulithi of Micronesia, the Ainu of northern Japan, the Twa of central Africa, and the Balinese of Indonesia have the same complexity of social patterns, cultural norms, and symbolic meaningfulness as do more familiar cultures such as the French, Germans, Chinese, and Americans. Each culture, in a sense, represents an alternative pattern of human experience with its own essential structural and functional integrity. Cross-cultural research shows anthropologists broad regularities in human actions and thought. Causal relationships among demographic variables, modes of subsistence, familial organizations, and belief systems have been established by anthropologists. The anthropological view has considerable temporal and spatial depth. It is precisely this cross-cultural perspective and the Rey concept of *culture* that have enabled many anthropologists to understand that AIDS is more than just another disease. It is, in a sense, a microcosm for understanding and synthesizing the human condition. This anthropological perspective is, of course, also shared by many people who are not anthropologists.

International and domestic AIDS policy formulation requires a very broad understanding of the human condition. Anthropology, perhaps more than most other academic disciplines, is well situated, with its propensity to maintain a global and evolutionary perspective, to begin to play a central and indispensable role in the development of intelligently constructed international and domestic AIDS policies.

The struggle against AIDS requires all relevant scientific and social scientific disciplines to work fervently to combat this insidious epidemic. Anthropology is beginning to now do its fair share.

On an even broader level, perhaps no other event has brought together so many different kinds of scientists and practitioners than has the AIDS crisis. Medicine, law, social services, education, biological sciences, social and behavioral sciences, ethics, politics, and other areas of human endeavor have played an integral role in understanding and controlling the development of this global pandemic. It is a war that must be fought on all fronts to be won. It is through this interdisciplinary approach that AIDS can most successfully be confronted. And it is precisely through this confrontation that we are beginning to learn more about ourselves as a most unique and very special species.

## NOTE

An earlier version of this chapter was presented at the V International Conference on AIDS, Montreal, June 1989. I would like to thank Dr. Ronald Prineas, Dr. Frank Stitt, and Dr. Dooley Worth for their comments.

## REFERENCES

Carrier, Joseph M., and J.R. Magana. (1989). "Mexican and Mexican-American Male Sexual Behavior and the Spread of AIDS in California," National Institutes of Health Workshop on AIDS and Sexual Behavior, May 18–19.

Trotter, Robert T., II. (1988). "Comments on Ethnographic Research Design: a Guide for DAAR–2," unpublished paper.

# Index

Africa: HIV infection in, 2, 16–17, 46; protozoal infection in, 47; retroviruses in, 14; sexually transmitted diseases in, 50

African swine fever virus, 48–49; mutated form in humans, 48

AIDS: cause of rapid spread, 1–2; CDC-defined, 12; classification by researchers, 14; definition in relation to other diseases, 13; "disease" versus "illness," 55, 59, 64; education/research in the Third World, 6–7; effect on gay culture, 4, 46–47; moral judgments on, 3, 38, 55–56, 60; nomenclature, 138; policy and law, 20–22, 30, 33–36, 49, 59–60, 69, 87; possible origin, 1–2, 11, 15–16, 48, 58, 68; research implications, 15

AIDS-related complex, 12

American Indians: blame/responsibility by, 144; use of English loan words by, 143

Anthropology, 128 n.1, 170; activities/projects, 205; associations, 86, 205; broad perspective provided by, 207–8; cooperation with/of other disciplines, 51, 208; ethnography, 205–6; other ethnography studies, 206–7; responsibilities of, 86, 207; use of, in international studies, 207

AZT (azidothymidine or Retrovir), 187

Bisexual men: estimated U.S. population, 3; in Haiti, 72–73; HIV infection in the United States of, 160

Blacks: deviant behavior in, 122, 124; disease in, 121; homosexuality in, 121–22

Black women: condom use with, 123; denial of risk for AIDS by, 126; factors shaping gender relations of, 122–24; influence of religion on, 123–25, 130 n.31; intravenous drug use by, 124–25; male sexual partners of, 123, 125; myths/sterotyping of, 122–23

Blame/responsibility, 2; by American Indians, 144; of Haitians, 68, 72, 83; of homosexuals, 172–73, 180; of people with AIDS, 30, 32–35, 41–42, 113; by society, 15, 32–34, 41, 58, 112, 125, 150, 167

Blood: contaminated donations, 2, 34; donations by Haitians, 70; donors in Rwanda, 46; received by Haitians, 72;

## ABOUT THE EDITOR AND CONTRIBUTORS

DOUGLAS A. FELDMAN, Ph.D., is a medical anthropologist and an Associate Professor in the Department of Epidemiology and Public Health at the University of Miami School of Medicine. He conducted AIDS social research in New York City beginning in 1982, was the first anthropologist to do AIDS research in Africa in 1985, and was the founding director of AIDS Center of Queens County (an AIDS service, counseling and educational organization) in New York City from 1986–88. He founded the AIDS and Anthropology Research Group and cofounded the American Anthropological Association Task Force on AIDS. He is a member of the Scientific and Technical Advisory Committee to the International Forum for AIDS Research of the Institute of Medicine. Since 1989, he has been developing AIDS research projects for South Florida, Thailand, and Africa. Dr. Feldman coedited *The Social Dimensions of AIDS: Method and Theory* (Praeger, 1986).

SOPHIE DAY, Ph.D., is a Research Associate in the Department of Anthropology at the London School of Economics and an Honorary Research Fellow in Academic Department of Public Health, St. Mary's Hospital Medical School.

PAUL FARMER, M.D., Ph.D., is an Instructor in the Department of Social Medicine at Harvard University, and has conducted fieldwork in rural Haiti.

NORRIS G. LANG, Ph.D., is an Associate Professor of Anthropology at the University of Houston, and an Associate Clinical Practitioner at the New Counseling Center in Houston, Texas.

WILLIAM L. LEAP, Ph.D., is an anthropological linguist and an Associate Professor of Anthropology at the American University in Washington, D. C. and has conducted research on the scoiolinguistics of AIDS.

S. C. McCOMBIE, Ph.D., is a medical anthropologist with interests in the evolution of infectious disease, currently conducting research on AIDS in Africa and the Caribbean through the Center for International, Health, and Development Communication at the University of Pennsylvania.

PETER M. NARDI, Ph.D., is a Professor of Sociology at Pitzer College of the

Claremont Colleges and an editor of a special issue of *California Sociologist* on AIDS.

JULIET A. NIEHAUS, Ph.D., C.S.W., is both an anthropologist and clinical social worker who teaches social work in the Department of Sociology and Anthropology at Wagner College in Staten Island, New York.

MICHAEL D. QUAM, Ph.D., M.P.H., Professor of Anthrology and Health Services Administration at Sangamon State University, is active in community health organizing and education, and a consultant to the Illinois Department of Public Health.

CHRISTOPHER C. TAYLOR, Ph.D., is a Mellon Instructor in the Social Sciences at the University of Chicago, and specializes in the study of Rwandan popular medicine.

DOOLEY WORTH, Ph.D., is Senior Corporate Health Project Advisor for the President of the New York Health and Hospitals Corporation, and has conducted research on women and AIDS.